# Psychiatric Mental Health Nursing: An Update

*Editor*

DEBORAH ANTAI-OTONG

# NURSING CLINICS
# OF NORTH AMERICA

www.nursing.theclinics.com

*Consulting Editor*
STEPHEN D. KRAU

June 2016 • Volume 51 • Number 2

**ELSEVIER**

1600 John F. Kennedy Boulevard • Suite 1800 • Philadelphia, Pennsylvania, 19103-2899

http://www.theclinics.com

**NURSING CLINICS OF NORTH AMERICA Volume 51, Number 2**
**June 2016 ISSN 0029-6465, ISBN-13: 978-0-323-44654-9**

Editor: Kerry Holland
Developmental Editor: Casey Jackson

*Nursing Clinics of North America* (ISSN 0029-6465) is published quarterly by Elsevier Inc., 360 Park Avenue South, New York, NY 10010-1710. Months of issue are March, June, September, and December. Periodicals postage paid at New York, NY and additional mailing offices. Subscription price per year is, $155.00 (US individuals), $447.00 (US institutions), $275.00 (international individuals), $545.00 (international institutions), $220.00 (Canadian individuals), $545.00 (Canadian institutions), $100.00 (US students), and $135.00 (international students). To receive student/resident rate, orders must be accompanied by name of affiliated institution, date of term, and the signature of program/residency coordinator on institution letterhead. Orders will be billed at individual rate until proof of status is received. Foreign air speed delivery is included in all *Clinics* subscription prices. All prices are subject to change without notice. **POSTMASTER:** Send address changes to *Nursing Clinics*, Elsevier Health Sciences Division, Subscription Customer Service, 3251 Riverport Lane, Maryland Heights, MO 63043. **Customer Service: Telephone: 1-800-654-2452** (U.S. and Canada); **1-314-447-8871 (outside U.S. and Canada). Fax: 1-314-447-8029. E-mail: journalscustomerservice-usa@elsevier.com** (for print support) and **journalsonlinesupport-usa@elsevier.com** (for online support).

*Nursing Clinics of North America* is covered in *EMBASE/Excerpta Medica, MEDLINE/PubMed (Index Medicus), Social Sciences Citation Index, Current Contents, ASCA, Cumulative Index to Nursing, RNdex Top 100,* and Allied Health Literature and International Nursing Index (INI).

# Contributors

## CONSULTING EDITOR

**STEPHEN D. KRAU, PhD, RN, CNE**
Associate Professor, Vanderbilt University School of Nursing, Nashville, Tennessee

## EDITOR

**DEBORAH ANTAI-OTONG, MS, APRN, PMHCNS-BC, FAAN**
Continuous Readiness Officer and Mental Health Consultant, Department of Veterans Affairs, Veterans Integrated Service Networks-(VISN-17), Arlington, Texas

## AUTHORS

**DEBORAH ANTAI-OTONG, MS, APRN, PMHCNS-BC, FAAN**
Continuous Readiness Officer and Mental Health Consultant, Department of Veterans Affairs, Veterans Integrated Service Networks-(VISN-17), Arlington, Texas

**LINDA FUNK BARLOON, MS(N), RN, PMHNP-BC, PMHCNS-BC**
Psychiatric Nurse Practitioner, Neurological Institute, The Houston Methodist Hospital, Houston, Texas

**ANDREA C. BOSTROM, PhD, PMHCNS-BC, RN**
Professor, Kirkhof College of Nursing, Grand Valley State University, Grand Rapids, Michigan

**REBECCA CLOUGH, MSN, APRN, PMHCNS-BC**
Associate Chief Nurse, Outpatient Mental Health, Salt Lake City VA Health Care System, Salt Lake City, Utah

**JULIE P. DUNNE, MSN, RN, PMHNP-BC**
University Fellow, Boston College Wm. F. Connell School of Nursing, Chestnut Hill, Massachusetts

**COURTNEY J. GIVENS, PharmD**
Clinical Pharmacy Specialist, Mental Health, VA North Texas Health Care System, Dallas, Texas

**WANDA HILLIARD, MBA, APRN, PMHNP-BC, RN, DNP**
University of Texas Medical Branch, Correctional Managed Care, Galveston, Texas

**LISA JENSEN, DNP, APRN, PMHCNS-BC**
Associate Director Workforce and Leadership, Office of Nursing Services, Veteran's Health Administration, Washington, DC

**RICHARD L. JOHN Jr, MSN, PMHNP-BC, FNP-BC**
Department of Veterans Affairs-Greater Los Angeles, Los Angeles, California

**MEREDITH R. KELLS, MSN, RN, CPNP**
University Fellow, Boston College Wm. F. Connell School of Nursing, Chestnut Hill, Massachusetts

**CINDY PARSONS, DNP, ARNP, PMHNP-BC, FAANP**
Associate Professor of Nursing, University of Tampa, Tampa, Florida

**DEE DEE PATRICK, MS, RN, CARN**
Frankfort, Illinois

**JEFFERY RAMIREZ, PhD, PMHNP**
Associate Professor, Department of Nursing and Human Physiology, Gonzaga University; Psychiatric Nurse Practitioner, Mann-Grandstaff VA Medical Center, Spokane, Washington

**CAROLYN SEEGANNA, MS, RN, CNS, ANP**
Department of Veterans Affairs, Mat-Su Community Based Outpatient Clinic, Wasilla, Alaska

**KRISTINE THEIS, FNP, MSN, RN**
Chief Nurse Behavioral Health, Member of ONS Mental Health Field Advisory Committee, Boise VAMC, Boise, Idaho

**BARBARA E. WOLFE, PhD, RN, PMHCNS-BC, FAAN**
Associate Dean for Research and Professor, Boston College Wm. F. Connell School of Nursing, Chestnut Hill, Massachusetts

**MICHELE L. ZIMMERMAN, MA, PMHCNS-BC**
Finney Zimmerman Psychiatric Associates PLC, Virginia Beach, Virginia; Associate Professor Emerita, Psychiatric Nursing, Old Dominion University, Norfolk, Virginia

# Contents

Understanding and treating mental illness has improved in many ways as a result of the fast pace of technological advances. The technologies that have the greatest potential impact are those that (1) increase the knowledge of how the brain functions and changes based on interventions, (2) have the potential to personalize interventions based on understanding genetic factors of drug metabolism and pharmacodynamics, and (3) use information technology to provide treatment in the absence of an adequate mental health workforce. Technologies are explored for psychiatric nurses to consider. Psychiatric nurses are encouraged to consider the experiences of psychiatric patients, including poor health, stigmatization, and suffering.

There are major legal issues that affect psychiatric nursing and guidelines for practicing in a legal and responsible manner. Advances in understanding of psychiatric conditions and developments in how nurses care for psychiatric patients result in changes in regulations, case law, and policies that govern nursing practice. Professional development, keeping abreast of current research and literature regarding clinical practice and trends, and involvement in professional organizations are some of the ways that psychiatric nurses can meet the challenges of their profession.

Anxiety disorders are among the most prevalent and disabling psychiatric disorders. Patients and their families have a plethora of evidence-based treatment options to manage these potentially incapacitating and costly disorders. Nurses in various settings can assess symptoms of anxiety disorder and initiate or refer patients for treatment. Families play a critical role in treatment planning and must be part of the health care team. Primary nursing interventions must be person centered and recovery based to ensure accurate diagnosis, initiation of appropriate person-centered treatment, and facilitate an optimal level of functioning and quality of life.

Patients with acute psychosis often present to emergency departments. Management of acute agitation and psychosis can be a challenge for the staff. Medical stabilization, appropriate assessment, and diagnosis are important. Verbal de-escalation and other psychosocial interventions are helpful in creating a safe and therapeutic environment. Psychiatric and emergency room nurses are poised to treat patients presenting with acute psychosis and must be knowledgeable of evidence-based approaches to treat these complex disorders.

Attention deficit hyperactivity disorder (ADHD) is a common neurodevelopmental disorder in children, adolescents, and adults, with a prevalence estimated from 5% to 7% across cultures and approximately 2% to 5% in adults. This lifelong disorder challenges nurses to understand the basis of ADHD, analyze symptoms, differentiate coexisting disorders, gather health information from varied sources, and implement person-centered multimodal treatment. Nurses are poised to plan, and work with patients, families, and teachers in the community and school systems to optimize academic and occupational performance and improve quality of life. Pharmacotherapy, psychoeducation, and behavioral therapies are strong components of multimodal treatment planning.

Eating disorders are chronic psychiatric illnesses with significant medical complications, psychological distress, and psychiatric comorbidity. Although many patients are treated on an outpatient basis, inpatient care for the more severely ill hospitalized patient can be challenging given the severity of illness and concurrent issues requiring intervention. This article provides an overview of the clinical characteristics of eating disorders typically seen for inpatient care, focusing primarily on anorexia nervosa and bulimia nervosa, and the associated key areas for nursing assessment, diagnoses, and plan of care during hospitalization.

Dual diagnosis is a prevalent and serious health problem. These disorders challenge psychiatric mental health and addiction nurses to treat 2 distinct disorders. Despite advances in the treatment of these disorders, there remains a void in the ideal approach. This article offers psychiatric nurses opportunities to improve their expertise in the identification of vulnerable or high-risk populations by using integrated screening and brief interventions to discern treatment options. Patients who require comprehensive treatment to stabilize 1 or both disorders further challenge nurses to have a basic understanding of the powerful effects of substance use on psychiatric conditions and vice versa.

This article examines the challenges faced by adolescents and their families as the young person matures into adulthood. Crises are the result of unpredictable situations or events that overwhelm the individual or individuals and render their resources and coping skills ineffective in mediating the stress. Crises can be situational, maturational, or adventitious. Nurses of all specialties may encounter the individual or family in crisis and need to provide crisis interventions services while assisting them to access the services of a skilled mental health professional.

As the population ages, nurses in various clinical settings must identify high-risk groups that are vulnerable to delirium and dementia. They also must be able to provide psychosocial and pharmacologic interventions that promote comfort and safety for patients and their families experiencing these distressful medical conditions. Efforts to facilitate health resolution and restore the patient and caregivers to an optimal level of functioning must be priorities.

Suicide remains a major public health issue. There have been more than 40,000 deaths by suicide in 2014. Understanding both the neuroscience and psychological development is key for nursing care so adequate interventions and treatment strategies are developed when working with people thinking about suicide. It is critical to assess and recognize risk and protective factors to ensure patient safety. The older adult, children, and adolescent populations remain vulnerable to suicide. A discussion regarding the psychiatric, psychosocial, and treatment considerations for these populations is included. An overview of communication, suicide assessment, and safety planning is discussed.

This article discusses a psychosocial recovery and rehabilitation recovery model that uses an intensive case management approach. The approach offers an interdisciplinary model that integrates pharmacotherapy, social skills training, cognitive remediation, family involvement, and community integration. This evidence-based plan of care instills hope and nurtures one's capacity to learn and improve function and quality of life. It is cost-effective and offers psychiatric nurses opportunities to facilitate symptomatic remission, facilitate self-efficacy, and improve communication and social cognition skills. Nurses in diverse practice settings must be willing to plan and implement innovative treatment models that provide seamless mental health care across the treatment continuum.

Borderline personality disorder (BPD) is a complex, serious, and high-cost psychiatric disorder. The high prevalence of patients with BPD and co-occurring depression, eating disorders, and substance-use disorders in primary care and mental health settings contribute to their high use of resources in these practice settings. Regardless of treatment challenges associated with BPD, researchers suggest a more positive outlook in the treatment of this complex psychiatric condition. This article focuses on areas in which nurses can strengthen their understanding of underpinnings and multimodal approaches, assess the patient's immediate needs, and manage distressful emotional states and impulsivity.

The advent of psychotropic medications in the 1950s greatly impacted the practice of psychiatry. Since then, efforts have been made to produce effective medications with few side effects (SEs) or adverse drug reactions (ADRs). Newer psychotropics have been developed but are not without risk. ADRs and SEs can lead to medication noncompliance, morbidity, and mortality. In many cases, ADRs can be prevented and common SEs relieved through proper interventions. Nursing interventions are vital to improving patient safety and outcomes in mental health populations. This article discusses ADRs and SEs of antipsychotics, antidepressants, mood stabilizers, and stimulants.

Although trauma exposure is common, few people develop acute and chronic psychiatric disorders. Those who develop posttraumatic stress disorder likely have coexisting psychiatric and physical disorders. Psychiatric nurses must be knowledgeable about trauma responses, implement evidence-based approaches to conduct assessments, and create safe environments for patients. Most researchers assert that trauma-focused cognitive-behavioral approaches demonstrate the most efficacious treatment outcomes. Integrated approaches, offer promising treatment options. This article provides an overview of clinical factors necessary to help the trauma survivor begin the process of healing and recovery and attain an optimal level of functioning.

Richard L. John Jr and Deborah Antai-Otong

Mood disorders have a high incidence of coexisting psychiatric, substance use, and physical disorders. When these disorders are unrecognized and left untreated, patients are likely to have a reduced life expectancy and experience impaired functional and psychosocial deficits and poor quality of life. Psychiatric nurses are poised to address the needs of these patients through various approaches. Although the ideal approach for mood disorders continues to be researched, there is a compilation of data showing that integrated models of treatment that reflect person-centered, strength, and recovery-based principles produce positive clinical outcomes.

# NURSING CLINICS OF NORTH AMERICA

**THE CLINICS ARE AVAILABLE ONLINE!**
Access your subscription at:
www.theclinics.com

# Foreword

# Patients with Mental Health Issues Transcend Centralized Care Settings

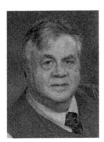

Stephen D. Krau, PhD, RN, CNE
*Consulting Editor*

Among the many trends in health care and nursing, one of the most dynamic areas of our profession is the area of psychiatric/mental health nursing. This may be a reflection of broader current issues and trends in the psychiatric well-being standards and treatments for our society. However, there are clear trends that have affected the changes in how Americans treat those with psychiatric issues. Over the last several decades, the location of psychiatric treatment has shifted from hospitals, or tertiary settings, to community settings, or primary settings.[1] With the "deinstitutionalization" of psychiatric patients, the responsibility and settings for care shifted to community agencies and settings that were not fully prepared for this role. As a result, the deinstitutionalization of these patients who are symptomatic was for all practical purposes a transinstutionalization of patients to other institutions such as general hospitals, nursing homes, half-way homes.[2]

Transinstitutionalization not only demonstrates the connectedness among institutional settings[3] but also indicates that nurses caring for psychiatric patients are no longer limited to specific settings. As it is common to see psychiatric issues associated with more "physical" comorbidities among patients admitted for nonpsychiatric issues, the likelihood of a nurse caring for patients with a psychiatric diagnosis increases drastically. To meet the needs of these patients, and to provide care that is holistic or complete, nurses are tasked with the responsibility of incorporating psychiatric issues and linkages to physical problems into a comprehensive plan of care. The need for learning about mental health issues in actuality transcends the boundaries in patient typology that has been created and promulgated by the health care system and nursing education.

There is much discussion about the psychological problems associated with our aging population. Some of the articles in this issue address these issues. What is

Nurs Clin N Am 51 (2016) xi–xii
http://dx.doi.org/10.1016/j.cnur.2016.04.002
0029-6465/16/$ – see front matter © 2016 Published by Elsevier Inc.

equally important is the increase of overall prescriptions but particularly the increase of psychotropic prescriptions that are written for children and adolescents. The growing trend is well documented.[4] This alone indicates a societal change in the distribution of thought and diagnoses of psychiatric disorders. Along with the increasing numbers of prescriptions and prescribers, a decentralized approach to providing care for psychiatric patients of any age poses the potential for miscommunication, lack of coordination, and lack of understanding about patients with psychiatric issues.

Stephen D. Krau, PhD, RN, CNE
Vanderbilt University School of Nursing
461 21st Avenue South
Nashville, TN, 37240, USA

E-mail address:
steve.krau@vanderbilt.edu

## REFERENCES

1. Bowersox NW, Szymanski BJ, McCarthy JF. Associations between psychiatric inpatient bed supply and the prevalence of serious mental illness in Veterans Affairs nursing homes. Am J Public Health 2013;103(7):1325–31.
2. Geller JL. The last half-century of psychiatric services as reflected in psychiatric services. Psychiatr Serv 2000;51(1):41–67.
3. Prins SJ. Does transinstitutionalization explain the overrepresentation of people with serious mental illnesses in the criminal justice system? Community Ment Health J 2011;47(6):716–22.
4. Steinhausen HC. Recent international trends in psychotropic medication prescriptions for children and adolescents. Eur Child Adolesc Psychiatry 2015;24(6): 635–40.

# Preface

# Psychiatric Mental Health Nursing: An Update

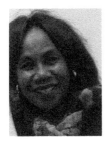

Deborah Antai-Otong, MS, APRN, PMHCNS-BC, FAAN
*Editor*

It is a great privilege to be the guest editor of *Nursing Clinics of North America*'s Psychiatric Mental Health Nursing updated issue. Since the first issue was published in 2003, there has been a plethora of scientific evidence from neurobiological research, technological advances, neuroimaging studies, and pharmacotherapies that target complex brain regions, neural pathways, neuroendocrine processes, and gender and genetic underpinnings that contribute to various psychiatric disorders. There has also been an explosion of evidence-based psychotherapeutic and pharmacologic approaches that address the needs of clients presenting with psychiatric and coexisting medical conditions. Combining this evidence emphasizes the significance of person-centered and holistic treatment and recovery-based models that instill hope, resilience, and strength and facilitate family involvement and community integration. As more and more clients with psychiatric disorders seek treatment in vast health care settings, including primary care, it imperative for nurses in all settings to assess and address the complex needs of this population.

The foremost strength of this issue is its expansive emphasis and synthesis of empirical data into psychiatric mental health nursing practice. Psychiatric nurses and nonpsychiatric nurses will find this updated issue refreshing and useful in their assessment, diagnosis, and implementation of person-centered mental health care. The initial section focuses on technological advances and the art of psychiatric mental health nursing and legal aspects of psychiatric nursing when caring for the client with a psychiatric disorder. The following sections provide updates on the treatment of mood disorders, acute psychosis, attention-deficit hyperactivity disorder, substance-use disorders, eating disorders, and borderline personality disorder. Followed by sections focusing on the care of adolescents and families in crisis, geriatric psychiatric emergencies, suicide, psychosocial recovery and rehabilitation, and adverse drug reactions, along with a new article on trauma survivors. Each article integrated evidence-based and recovery and person-centered approaches, including pharmacotherapy and psychotherapeutic

Nurs Clin N Am 51 (2016) xiii–xiv
http://dx.doi.org/10.1016/j.cnur.2016.04.001
0029-6465/16/$ – see front matter © 2016 Published by Elsevier Inc.

nursing.theclinics.com

modalities, such as psychotherapy, psychoeducation, family involvement, and psychosocial rehabilitation.

This updated issue of *Nursing Clinics of North America* incorporates the expertise of advanced practice psychiatric mental health registered nurses who were invited to update their articles from the previous issue along with several new authors. This compilation of authors reflects diverse practice settings and universities who willingly shared their expertise in the care of individuals with psychiatric disorders. This issue also reflects the unique contributions of psychiatric mental health nursing and its significant contributions in health promotion, resilience, and recovery across the lifespan.

Deborah Antai-Otong, MS, APRN, PMHCNS-BC, FAAN
Department of Veterans Affairs
Veterans Integrated Service Networks (VISN-17)
2301 East Lamar Boulevard
Arlington, TX 76006, USA

E-mail address:
Deborah.Antai-Otong@va.gov

# Technological Advances in Psychiatric Nursing

## An update

Andrea C. Bostrom, PhD, PMHCNS-BC, RN

### KEYWORDS

- Brain imaging technology • Health information technology • Pharmacogenetics
- Telepsychiatry • Computer based psychiatric interventions

### KEY POINTS

- Brain imaging, genetics, and information technology are areas within which considerable knowledge is being generated that can be applied to psychiatric nursing.
- Several technologies have been used to explore brain functioning as a result of psychiatric symptoms and hypothesized treatment interventions.
- Pharmacogenetics supports exploration of personalized medication treatment; however, at this time it is limited to understanding the genetics associated with the metabolism of psychiatric drugs and genetic contributions to easily measured effects, for example, metabolic changes.
- Health information technology (HIT) has potential to provide better measures and assessment of quality outcomes in psychiatric care and to explore innovative methods to provide psychiatric treatment over the Internet or using other types of applications. Although there are issues of expense and privacy for mental health providers, the creative use of HIT may address the critical workforce limitations.

### INTRODUCTION

Traditionally, mental health and psychiatric care has made minimal use of technology. A little more than a decade ago, the technological advances that affected modern mental health nursing were described.[1] These advances highlighted the wonders of brain scanning that gave information without waiting for autopsy results, the emerging efforts of genetic explorations that held hope for creating more targeted treatments for mental illness, and the creative manipulations of medications to improve effectiveness

This article is an update of an article previously published in Nursing Clinics of North America, Volume 38, Issue 1, March 2003.

Disclosure Statement: None.

Kirkhof College of Nursing, Grand Valley State University, 301 Michigan Street NE, Grand Rapids, MI 49503-3314, USA

E-mail address: bostroma@gvsu.edu

and diminish unpleasant side effects. Since the publication of the original article, several technological advances have changed health care and have stimulated ideas for improving treatment of people with mental illness. These advances include the successful sequencing of the human genome concurrent with the publication of the original article, the first iPhone in 2007 (C.A. Bostrom, personal communication, 2015), and the extensive implementation of electronic health records (EHRs) and other health information technologies.

## UPDATE ON TECHNOLOGIES DESCRIBED IN THE ORIGINAL ARTICLE
### Brain Scans/Imaging Technologies

Several neuroimaging technologies have been used for at least the past 2 decades to increase understanding of brain changes that occur with mental illness and its treatment. Prior to the use of these technologies, autopsies were the main method of examining brain structures. The problems with autopsies, however, were the difficulty determining the history of the disease and its treatment prior to an individual's death and the inability to determine concurrent information about behavior and brain function because the subject was no longer alive. On the other hand, neuroimaging techniques can be used with full knowledge of an individual's illness history, treatment history, and current state of illness and symptoms. These techniques have led to much clearer knowledge of which behaviors and behavioral deficits are connected to brain structures and activity. Neuroimaging is used for both research and clinical assessment.

Structural neuroimaging techniques include CT and MRI scanning. With CT and MRI scans, clinicians and researchers can examine the brain for changes in structure and for brain lesions. CT scans use x-rays to create a series of gray-scale pictures of the brain, with structures absorbing the most x-rays appearing the lightest (bone) and those absorbing the least appearing the darkest (cerebrospinal fluid). The gray matter and white matter of the brain are the most difficult to distinguish on CT scans. With MRIs, an image is created when the magnetic field in the MRI aligns the protons inside atoms in the brain and uses radio waves to disrupt the alignment and then measure the radio waves emitted by the protons as they return to alignment.[2] This results in a 3-D image that more clearly distinguishes the white matter and gray matter of the brain.

Functional imaging includes PET scans, single-photon emission CT (SPECT), and functional MRI (fMRI) scanning. PET scans create stunning colorful pictures of the brain showing overactivity or underactivity in brain regions based on glucose consumption and cerebral blood flow while the brain is at rest or while an individual does tasks. With SPECT, structural images created by the functioning of regional cerebral blood flow show deviations from symmetry (individuals essentially serve as their own controls) that can indicate pathology and distinguish among possible diagnoses with symptoms that are difficult to distinguish, for example, dementias.[3] An fMRI uses the magnetic field in a slightly different way from the MRI.[2] With an fMRI, the magnetic field takes advantage of the iron within oxygen-rich blood that rushes to an area in the brain activated by some task or stimulus. This results in an image of functional brain activity. fMRIs have become beneficial for research on brain function and behavior, such as anxiety, social functioning, dyslexia, and addictions.[2]

There are both benefits and challenges to using these scanning methodologies. The obvious benefits are their noninvasive methods that produce information to increase understanding of the normal brain and the impact of mental illness. That said, the equipment used for many of these scans can be intimidating. For MRIs in particular, an individual is required to lie very still in a tube that can feel claustrophobic while loud banging noises are produced during the test. The scan itself can take 20 to 40 minutes. With fMRIs, a special mask may be prepared for an individual to help with immobilizing the head, further adding to the sense of closeness. Individuals need to be prepared to use relaxation techniques, like deep breathing, to help manage any discomfort and anxiety. Education about the procedures is required. Because fMRIs are frequently used to test hypotheses about brain functioning, individuals may find the tasks that are projected on a screen within the equipment distracting enough to tolerate any discomfort with the procedure itself. Some individuals may require a trusted person to accompany them, even though that person is not allowed in the room while the test is done. PET, SPECT, and some CT scans may require the use of radioactive isotopes and radiation, thus limiting the frequency of their use. Most of these scanning technologies are also expensive.

Electroencephalography (EEG) is a noninvasive technology that continues to be used. EEGs record electrical activity of the brain using electrodes applied to the scalp. In the past decade, faster, smaller, and more powerful computers have facilitated a technical methodology called quantitative EEG (QEEG) analysis. With QEEG, an individual's EEG is converted to numbers that can then be compared with databases of EEGs of people with normal brain functioning for further analysis. This method is used to study many mental health disorders, including anxiety, depression, and autism.[4]

### Alternative Treatments/Biofeedback

Mindfulness interventions are supported for mental health conditions and for many stress-of-life situations. Many other alternative treatments continue to find support as treatment interventions, including yoga, meditation, aromatherapy, and acupressure/acupuncture. Although these interventions are decidedly low technology, they can be used with biofeedback. When biofeedback procedures are used, an individual learns to use relaxation methods from these various interventions while sensors for pulse, blood pressure, and skin temperature send data to monitors. Individuals use the visual feedback from the monitors to see the effectiveness of their relaxation methods. This combination of low-technology interventions with high-technology monitoring allows individuals to be successful without the monitors, at a later time, to lower stress, anxiety, and autonomic body responses.

### Genetics and Medications

The stress-diathesis model of many mental illnesses suggests that genetic factors lay down the susceptibility (the genotype) to mental illness whereas environmental stressors trigger the changes in symptoms and behaviors (the phenotype) consistent with mental illness. Environmental stressors describe a range of factors from the in utero environment to the broader environment. Genetic factors influence the development of mental illness; however, because there is not 100% heritability in families in which mental illnesses have emerged, the evidence for environmental factors is clear as well. Scientists also look to genetics to untangle individual responses to the medications used to treat mental illness in hopes of creating individualized and personalized medication treatment.

Pharmacogenetics is increasingly viable based on the successful sequencing of the human genome. The promising applications to mental health treatment are, however, limited. One area that has received considerable attention is related to the metabolism of drugs and the polymorphic variants of cytochrome P450 enzymes (discussed by Krau[5–7] in 3 recent articles). For example, 1 of these specific enzymes, CYP2D6, has been studied extensively in relationship to the metabolism of antidepressant medications.[8] Based on gene copies inherited, people can be categorized into poor, intermediate, extensive, or ultrarapid metabolizers. Poor metabolizers have slower clearance of drugs from the blood, are more likely to have adverse drug reactions at lower doses, and are more likely to stop taking the medication due to these reactions. At the other end of the spectrum, where metabolism is speeded up, the rapid removal of the drug from the blood results in less effectiveness and a need for a higher dose of medication. Unfortunately, tests to examine the variations of CYP450 variants have not fulfilled their promise to date because (1) genotyping has not been consistently associated with obvious symptoms, behaviors, and drug responses; (2) of their expense; and (3) results may take 2 or more weeks—well past the time when an acute decision about a medication must be made to treat distress caused by mental illness. Nevertheless, knowledge about people having genetic differences in metabolism of these drugs, in particular antidepressants, may help with clinical observations when people seem less compliant or less responsive to a drug.

Pharmacogenetic studies have focused on the pharmacodynamic aspects of psychiatric medication effectiveness as well. These studies include the genetic aspects of monoamine (dopamine, norepinephrine, and serotonin) transporters, monoamine metabolic enzymes, and monoamine receptors within the cells of the brain.[8]

Although genetic studies continue to hold promise for personalized medical treatment, there are problems with the broad application of the findings. Zhang and Malhotra[9] outline the problems with pharmacogenetics and antipsychotic drugs. One issue is that it is easier to associate genetic findings with easily measured symptoms or adverse drug reactions. For instance, antipsychotic-associated weight gain and clozapine-induced agranulocytosis can be measured reliably using body mass index and total fat mass for the former or absolute neutrophil count for the latter. Unfortunately, there are few measures of symptoms of psychotic disorders used reliably in practice. In research, the limited number of comprehensive and reliable measures of symptoms and behaviors inhibit effective phenotype assessment. Another issue is that prospective randomized clinical trials comparing people who are newly diagnosed with their illness would allow better comparisons of those with similar genotypes and their responses to selected medications and treatments. Unfortunately, current understanding about genotypes and drug responses is based on retrospective trials with large proportions of chronically ill patients. Correcting these and other issues would make pharmacogenetics more useful in clinical practice.

The technologies discussed at this point are used to understand the biological aspects of mental illnesses and their contribution to how people respond to treatment. Information technologies, which are increasingly used to deliver treatment, are discussed next.

## APPLICATIONS FOR COMPUTER TECHNOLOGIES

Multiple factors are driving efforts to develop and use computer technologies in mental health. The increasingly smaller and powerful computers, tablets, and smartphones make communication anywhere and everywhere a possibility. The well-documented shortage of mental health providers, particularly in rural and small town communities, calls for creative methods to effectively reach people outside of cities with large medical centers. Several treatment interventions, such as cognitive behavior therapy (CBT), that use paper-and-pencil activities, can be translated to virtual activities. Avatars can be created to talk to clients in a virtual conversation or to train therapists about communication patterns. Patient portals in EHRs can enhance communication between patients and providers. Creative use of portals and smartphone applications can allow monitoring of symptoms and the effectiveness and use of prescribed medications. These technologies add flexibility to the treatment of mental illness.

## Internet-Based Treatment

Computer-based and Internet-based psychotherapy treatments of depression and anxiety have been developed and used for many years. Wright and Wright[10] summarized some of the benefits of developing computerized tools to enhance psychotherapy. These benefits include decreasing costs while increasing accessibility of psychotherapy; increased engagement, self-help, and self-monitoring; psychoeducation; and collecting data that could be translated into outcome measures of treatment effectiveness. Wright and Wright also identified concerns about using computers and the Internet. These concerns include confidentiality, access to and capacity to use computers and the Internet, adequate orientation to the computer program, sufficient and regular updating of information within the program, and sufficient access to a clinician during and after use of the computerized program. Despite the ubiquitous use of computers, these benefits and concerns are still valid when considering the use of computer-based treatments.

CBT-computerized programs have been studied widely. Several meta-analyses of computerized CBT studies[11–14] have found support for the effectiveness of CBT delivered via computer and Internet. Several programs are commercially produced. These programs have differing numbers of modules and include a variety of multimedia approaches to deliver the content. The meta-analyses identified areas for further exploration. There is still a need to identify the type of patient and the specific diagnoses and symptoms that are best suited to computerized treatment. Most studies have been limited to adult populations, so effectiveness with children and adolescents needs to be studied. A notable issue that emerged from some of the studies is the level of support needed to avoid early dropout from the program and to maintain long-term effects. In the most recent meta-analysis,[13] therapist and/or administrative support was an important component of completion of the program and effectiveness of the intervention.

Gilbody and colleagues[15] compared depression treatment as usual in primary care with a commercially available computerized CBT treatment (Beating the Blues) and a free-to-use treatment (MoodGYM). In the United Kingdom (where this study was conducted), the National Institute of Health and Care Excellence guidelines include computerized CBT treatments. The findings from this clinical trial suggest little difference in overall effectiveness among the treatments. Gilbody and colleagues[15] also found that few of the subjects completed all the modules available in the computerized programs, even with regular telephone support from research assistants. One particular issue that participants expressed was the difficulty, while clinically depressed, to repeatedly log into the computer program; they wanted more clinical support.

Avatars are another intriguing computer application. Leff and colleagues[16] piloted the use of avatars to help individuals who experience persecutory auditory hallucinations. In their procedure, patients selected a face and voice from a computer program package to represent the voice they hear. They then participated in six 30-minute weekly sessions. During these sessions they sat in a chair facing a monitor on which the avatar was displayed. The therapist, sitting in another room, speaks both for the avatar in the selected voice and as the therapist in a normal voice (controlled by the therapist through the computer program). The therapist encourages the patient to interact with the avatar and oppose its statements. Over the course of the 6 weeks, the avatar becomes less persecutory and more supportive (as controlled by the therapist). The sessions were also recorded and transferred to a device so that the patient could listen to the sessions to strengthen control of the voice. Although not everyone in the trial completed the intervention (17 of 26 completed all sessions), the intervention was successful for those who participated. For a few, the impact was dramatic.

Avatars have also been developed for simulated experiences. The University of Southern California's Institute for Creative Technologies (ict.usc.edu) created "Ellie" using SimSensei. Ellie performs as a therapist using the MultiSense software. Ellie can be observed using the following link: https://www.youtube.com/watch?v=ejczMs6b1Q4. The explanation for how MultiSense is used can be observed with the following link: https://www.youtube.com/watch?v=_uYokWUSark. These creative uses of computer applications are examples of how technology can be used as innovative treatment methods for mental health.

## Telecommunications in Psychiatry

Managing psychiatric care from a distance due to workforce shortages and the inadequate geographic distribution of the workforce has been a major incentive to provide mental health care in unique ways. Although face-to-face meetings between patients and mental health providers are the typical means of providing treatment, several alternatives have been explored to overcome distance barriers. Many agencies without access to psychiatric services for diagnosis and medication prescription use Internet video-conferencing to provide these services to their clients. Telephone-administered CBT was compared with face-to-face treatment in 1 study.[17] These researchers found that fewer patients dropped out of treatment with the telephone-administered CBT, but patients maintained improvements better at 6 months in the face-to-face group. Asynchronous telepsychiatry assisted another group to provide care to Spanish-speaking patients more effectively.[18] Interviews of the Spanish-speaking patients were taped and securely stored for translation and analysis by a consulting psychiatrist. The investigators of this pilot study found they could provide cost-effective consultation in a more timely and convenient process by avoiding the need to coordinate a face-to-face interview between the consultant and the patient in the presence of a translator. Providers in another study used telepsychiatry to provide temporary psychiatric service coverage to a rural general hospital with a psychiatric unit.[19] These researchers found their application of telepsychiatry feasible and acceptable. These examples suggest that distances and shortages can be overcome by the thoughtful use of technology.

## Health Information Technology

HIT includes EHRs, personal health records, health information exchanges (HIEs), and smartphone applications.[20] HITs hold great promise to help coordinate and integrate health care for people with psychiatric diagnoses. Many people, especially those with diagnoses of depression and anxiety, receive their mental health care in primary care practices. Many people with severe and persistent mental illness have substantial needs to help manage chronic health conditions that result from lifestyle and treatment effects. The ability to use information technology for enhanced communication between primary care and psychiatric services has great potential to decrease patient suffering.

EHRs, in particular, have the potential to facilitate better communication, better coordination of care, and better patient outcomes in behavioral and mental health treatment. Several barriers, however, to broad implementation of EHRs exist. The most challenging barriers are financial issues, privacy issues, and lack of standardization of quality measures for psychiatric screening, assessment, and outcomes.[20] Most psychiatric conditions are treated outside of large hospitals within the public mental health system, by qualified providers who are not physicians, and in small practices. The costs of implementing and maintaining EHRs in these types of practices can be insurmountable. Mental health and substance abuse services also require greater efforts to protect privacy than the requirements established by the Health Insurance Portability and Accountability Act. For federally assisted substance abuse programs, release of sensitive information is regulated by 42 CFR Part 2, which requires signed consent to release information to any entity (including any subsequent release from the original requester).[21] In addition, regulations protecting personal health information vary from state to state. Finally, effective use of EHRs and other HITs require standardized measures for comparison of effectiveness and assessment of the meaningful use of this technology.

In terms of the cost of implementing EHRs, the Affordable Care Act and the Health Information Technology for Economic and Clinical Health ACT incentivized the adoption and use of EHRs for health care providers to help coordinate and improve patient care. These incentives have been successful for EHR adoption among office-based physicians and acute care hospitals. Although acute care hospitals with psychiatric inpatient units benefit from these incentives, outpatient mental health practices were largely ineligible. As a result, mental health practices lag behind the incentivized providers in the adoption of EHRs. Two solutions for this oversight are lobbying efforts for new legislative initiatives and increasing evidence-based integration of behavioral and primary care practices. At the least, support for and participation in demonstration projects from the Substance Abuse and Mental Health Services Administration and Health Resources and Services Administration can facilitate solutions to the financial barrier.

In an effort to address the issues of exchanging behavioral health information while providing the necessary privacy protections, pilot projects have been implemented in several states, including Alabama, Florida, Kentucky, Michigan, Nebraska, and New Mexico.[21] These pilot projects identified recommendations to educate and inform all health care providers and patients about the legislated privacy requirements for behavioral health data exchange, to create consent and disclosure forms (and redisclosure forms) that can be used by HIEs to improve health outcomes for psychiatric patients, and to make certain that behavioral health data are taken into consideration as broad-based HIEs are developed.

Personal health records, patient portals, and applications for mobile devices like smartphones are being explored for usefulness, feasibility, and acceptability to help patients monitor their daily lives, symptoms, and treatments. Smartphone applications are increasingly feasible because they are owned in increasing numbers, even among people with lower incomes and individuals with severe mental illness.[22] Studies of smartphone applications for people with severe mental illness have found support for their use.[23,24] To enhance acceptability and usefulness, recommendations include collaborating with people for whom the application is designed to facilitate ease of use, initiating educational and practice activities to help individuals be comfortable with the technology, and engaging clinical staff to facilitate their comfort in adding this method of treatment and monitoring to traditional interventions. As with EHRs and HIEs, the privacy and safety of the information contained and transferred using these devices are essential concerns.

## RELATIONSHIP BETWEEN NURSING AND TECHNOLOGY IN MENTAL HEALTH CARE AND TREATMENT

In the earlier article,[1] 2 basic questions were asked: Has the technology changed how people with mental illness are treated? and How do nurses influence and apply technology and technological findings to psychiatric nursing care? These questions are still relevant across all levels of practicing nurses, from those who work in inpatient and outpatient settings to advanced practice nurses, whether they are nurse practitioners or clinical nurse specialists. The questions, however, can be expanded: Has the quality of life of people with mental illness improved? and How can nurses use technology to improve the lives of people with mental illness? Nursing is intended to minister to people's responses to their illnesses. In this role, there may be helpful ways to apply knowledge from technology, and technology itself, to people's responses.

The technology that has discovered areas in the brain associated with symptoms of mental illness is both helpful and not helpful. The public and people with mental illness can now point to a brain disorder as the cause of their symptoms, which has the potential to diminish the stigma of mental illnesses because the behaviors are no longer looked at as caused by deviance and moral deficiency. Individuals with mental illness may, however, feel discouraged, because they see the brain disorder as a life sentence. Many hypotheses tested with fMRIs examine how brain activity can change as a result of treatment interventions. Specific findings of these studies can be applied by nurses. Understanding the brain-changing impact of interventions provides increased rationale to nursing roles that manage the inpatient environment, that help patients manage daily life in the community, and that give comprehensive and supportive treatment beyond just the administration and prescription of medications.

Medications, both old and new, have an important place in the treatment of mental illnesses. The efforts to understand how and where they work in the brain can be greatly enhanced by efforts to describe and categorize symptoms and behaviors in a more reliable way. Patients are better served when nurses work within an interdisciplinary team that uses reliable tools to identify and measure target symptoms and side effects displayed by an individual. Personalized and individualized pharmacologic treatment (the promise of pharmacogenetics) cannot be realized without this activity. Furthermore, on a day-to-day basis, reliable measures help assess the effects of drugs indicative of people with different metabolizing rates.

HIT holds great promise for health care in general, and for mental health, in particular. The significant barriers to HITs' use in mental health must, however, be overcome. Policy changes that will help with financing and implementing EHRs require advocates who are willing to be politically active and demand parity with practices that treat physical illness. HIT holds promise to help those who seek treatment of anxiety and depression from their primary care providers and to help those with severe mental illness to have their physical health better managed. The communication, coordination, and effectiveness of this crossover care, however, cannot be attained without integration of practice and purpose, and advocacy for the change. These systems require considerable efforts to develop measures of symptoms and outcomes for quality management, to develop procedures and forms to support the privacy needed to avoid the effects of social stigma, and to create incentives for mental health and primary care practitioners to work together.

The lives of many people with mental illness, regardless of type, are full of suffering. Probably the most important measure of the usefulness of technology is the degree to which the suffering is lifted. There is reason to be hopeful; equally, there are outcomes that are still beyond reach. Until people with severe mental illness live longer and healthier lives, have better connections with their families, and are less likely to be imprisoned instead of treated, these technologies are not bringing about the kind of changes people need. Until treatment of depression, anxiety, and substance abuse is more accessible in rural and small town communities, these technologies will have not brought the workforce to the people who need it. Until treatment, using the knowledge gained from technology and and using information technology for communication and coordination, attains personalized and individualized treatment of mental illness, there is still work to be done.

## SUMMARY

Scientific progress, knowledge, and technology seem to be moving faster than many can comprehend. These continue to be exciting times as more about the brain and how to treat people with mental illness is understood. Yet nurses must never forget the real and frightening experiences that come with many mental illnesses. Technology and science enhance the work of clinicians, yet it is important to remember the day-to-day experiences of people with mental illness. The comment that ended the article a decade ago is still applicable: "Nurses, who help people respond to their illnesses, must engage science and technology with curiosity and engage the person with empathy."[1(p8)]

## REFERENCES

1. Bostrom AC. Technologic advances in psychiatric nursing. Nurs Clin North Am 2003;38(1):1–8.
2. Clay RA. Functional magnetic resonance imaging: a new research tool. Washington, DC: American Psychological Association; 2007.
3. Amen DG, Trujillo M, Newberg A, et al. Brain SPECT imaging in complex psychiatric cases: an evidence-based, underutilized tool. Open Neuroimag J 2011;5: 40–8.
4. Neurodevelopment Center. Quantitative EEG. Available at: http://neuro developmentcenter.com/neurofeedback-2/qeeg/. Accessed November 23, 2015.
5. Krau SD. Cytochrome p450, part 1: what nurses need to know. Nurs Clin North Am 2013;48:671–80.
6. Krau SD. Cytochrome p450, part 2: what nurses need to know about the cytochrome p450 family systems. Nurs Clin North Am 2013;48:681–96.
7. Krau SD. Cytochrome p450 part 3: essential concepts and considerations. Nurs Clin North Am 2013;48:697–706.
8. Weizman S, Gonda X, Dome P, et al. Pharmacogenetics of antidepressive drugs: a way towards personalized treatment of major depressive disorder. Neuropsychopharmacol Hung 2012;14(2):87–101.
9. Zhang J-P, Malhotra AK. Pharmacogenetics of antipsychotics: recent progress and methodological issues. Expert Opin Drug Metab Toxicol 2013;9(2):183–91.
10. Wright JE, Wright AS. Computer-assisted psychotherapy. J Psychother Pract Res 1997;6:315–29.
11. Andersson G, Cuijpers P. Internet-based and other computerized psychological treatments for adult depression: a meta-analysis. Cogn Behav Ther 2009;38: 196–205.
12. Andrews G, Cuijpers P, Craske MG, et al. Computer therapy for the anxiety and depressive disorders is effective, acceptable and practical health care: a meta-analysis. PLoS One 2010;5:e13196.
13. Richards D, Richardson T. Computer-based psychological treatments for depression: a systematic review and meta-analysis. Clin Psychol Rev 2012;32:329–42.
14. Spek V, Cuijpers P, Nyklicek I, et al. Internet-based cognitive behavior therapy for symptoms of depression and anxiety: a meta-analysis. Psychol Med 2007;37: 319–28.

15. Gilbody S, Littlewood E, Hewitt C, et al. Computerized cognitive behavior therapy (cCBT) as treatment for depression in primary care (REEACT trial): large scale pragmatic randomized controlled trial. BMJ 2015;351:h5627.
16. Leff J, Williams G, Huckvale M, et al. Avatar therapy for persecutory auditory hallucinations: what is it and how does it work? Psychosis 2014;6:166–76.
17. Mohr DC, Ho J, Duffecy J, et al. Effect of telephone-administered vs face-to-face cognitive behavioral therapy on adherence to therapy and depression outcomes among primary care patients: a randomized trial. JAMA 2012;307:2278–85.
18. Yellowlees PM, Odor A, Iosif A-M, et al. Transcultural psychiatry made simple—asynchronous telepsychiatry as an approach to providing culturally relevant care. Telemed J E Health 2013;19(4):1–6.
19. Grady B, Singleton M. Telepsychiatry "coverage" to a rural inpatient psychiatric unit. Telemed J E Health 2011;17:603–8.
20. Miller JE, Glover RW, Gordon SY. Crossing the behavioral digital divide: the role of health information technology in improving care for people with serious mental illness in state mental health systems. Alexandria (VA): National Association of State Mental Health Program Directors; 2014.
21. Office of the National Coordinator for Health Technology. Behavioral health data exchange consortium: ONC state health policy consortium project: final report. Research Triangle Park, NC: RTI International; 2014.
22. Firth J, Cotter J, Torous J. Mobile phone ownership and endorsement of "mHealth" among people with psychosis: a meta-analysis of cross-sectional studies. Schizophr Bull 2015 [Epub ahead of print]. Available at: http://schizophreniabulletin.oxfordjournals.org. Accessed December 5, 2015.
23. Ben-Zeev D, Brenner CJ, Begale M, et al. Feasibility, acceptability, ad preliminary efficacy of a smartphone intervention for schizophrenia. Schizophr Bull 2014;40:1244–53.
24. Ennis L, Robotham D, Denis M, et al. Collaborative development of an electronic personal health record for people with severe and enduring mental health problems. BMS Psychiatry 2014;14:301.

# Legal Considerations of Psychiatric Nursing Practice

Linda Funk Barloon, MS(N), RN, PMHNP-BC, PMHCNS-BC[a],*,
Wanda Hilliard, MBA, APRN, PMHNP-BC, RN, DNP[b]

## KEYWORDS

- Confidentiality • Informed consent • Civil commitment • Liability

## KEY POINTS

- There are major legal issues that affect psychiatric nursing and guidelines for practicing in a legal and responsible manner.
- Advances in understanding of psychiatric conditions and developments in how nurses care for psychiatric patients result in changes in regulations, case law, and policies that govern nursing practice.
- Professional development, keeping abreast of current research and literature regarding clinical practice and trends, and involvement in professional organizations are some of the ways that psychiatric nurses can meet the challenges of their profession.

## INTRODUCTION

The current landscape of health care requires that psychiatric nurses have a wide breadth of knowledge to practice in a responsible and legal manner. The emphasis on participation of informed patients and families within a recovery model, expanding costs and efforts to contain costs, and the goal of exclusively electronic records all add to the demand for knowledgeable nurses. For psychiatric nursing in particular, continuing advances in understanding of mental illness, genomics that relate to mental illness, and debates about patient rights versus societal safety are factors that have an impact on care. With the evolution of psychiatric care, the definition of legal practice also evolves over time. Psychiatric nurses are held accountable to practice according to current laws, regulations, and standards. This article briefly reviews the major legal issues that affect psychiatric nursing practice today.

This article is an update of an article previously published in Nursing Clinics of North America, Volume 38, Issue 1, March 2003.
The authors have no conflict of interest to disclose.
[a] The Houston Methodist Hospital, 6560 Fannin Street, Suite 944, Houston, TX 77030, USA;
[b] University of Texas Medical Branch, Correctional Managed Care, Galveston, TX, USA
* Corresponding author.
E-mail address: lbarloon@houstonmethodist.org

Nurs Clin N Am 51 (2016) 161–171
http://dx.doi.org/10.1016/j.cnur.2016.01.002
0029-6465/16/$ – see front matter © 2016 Elsevier Inc. All rights reserved.

nursing.theclinics.com

## STANDARDS FOR LEGAL PSYCHIATRIC NURSING PRACTICE

Legal parameters for practice are established through a variety of sources. Many measures exist against which a nurse's practice can be judged. State boards of nursing govern the scope of practice within a given state. Federal and state statues direct practice; for example, virtually all states have laws outlining the reporting of child and elder abuse. Case law (ie, legal findings related to particular court cases) also sets precedence for legal practice; for example, the Tarasoff case of the mid-1970s set a standard of the duty to protect third parties against harm that has become the benchmark in subsequent cases in other states. The Centers for Medicare and Medicare Services (CMS) sets stringent regulations for organizations that receive federal funding; for example, regulations define acceptable inpatient staff-to-patient ratios and proper training and use of seclusion and restraint. The Joint Commission is another body that sets rigorous standards for institutions that seek accreditation.[1] The Health Insurance Portability and Accountability Act of 1996 (HIPAA) is responsible for setting national standards for the security of a patient's electronic health information. All nurses are legally responsible for understanding the rules and regulations that govern this federal legislation.

Psychiatric nurses look to professional nursing organizations to define safe and acceptable practice through published standards. The American Nurses Association, utilizing a task force made of members of the American Psychiatric Nurses Association (APNA) and the International Society of Psychiatric-Mental Health Nurses (ISPN), published the revised of *Psychiatric-Mental Health Nursing: Scope and Standards of Practice*[2] in 2014. This comprehensive document outlines levels of psychiatric nursing practice and identifies specific standards of practice for nursing activities and criteria for measuring the standards.

Key changes in the *Psychiatric-Mental Health Nursing: Scope and Standards of Practice* include

- Emphasis on a recovery model with consumer participation in all aspects of treatment
- Paradigm shift toward prevention with psychiatric nurses promoting protective factors and environments and providing early screening and intervention
- Meeting the challenges of providing mental health care in integrated health care systems[3]

Similarly, the APNA and ISPN also have published standards that guide practice. Involvement in professional organizations can help nurses keep informed of current published standards as well as other issues.

Finally, developments in clinical practice guide legal practice. Advances in the study of the brain and behavior, neurochemical processes, new medications, the field of genetics, and the field of psychiatric nursing are constantly expanding.[3] Psychiatric nurses also continue to develop interviewing skills and therapeutic techniques. In addition to the foundation of knowledge and skills attained through basic nursing preparation, psychiatric nurses should remain current in clinical areas through participating in educational programs and reviewing the literature.

## PATIENT RIGHTS AND NURSING RESPONSIBILITIES
### Least Restrictive Alternative: Seclusion and Restraint

The use of seclusion and restraints is strictly regulated and psychiatric nurses are mandated to minimize if not eliminate the use of seclusion and restraint in psychiatric settings in the United States. Health care agency policies and governmental agencies and psychiatric organizations provide stringent guidelines that dictate the use of these treatment options. Restraint is defined as restricting a patient from moving freely by holding or by use of a device. Seclusion is preventing a patient from leaving a confined area or room.[4]

Psychiatric nurses must be knowledgeable about the potential physical as well as psychological injury to patients that may occur with seclusion and restraint use. An agency's philosophy on restraint use and the organizational culture may influence how patients are managed and may serve to reduce the incidence of seclusion and restraints. Decisions regarding the use of seclusion or restraint require complex and rapid nursing assessment to consider alternatives and to determine whether these measures are the only safe option. The decision to initiate seclusion and restraint is made only to keep patients and staff safe in emergency situations.[5]

The CMS sets guidelines, which apply to all health care agencies accepting Medicare and Medicaid payments, for the use of seclusion and restraint. Within 1 hour of the initiation of seclusion or restraint, a face-to-face evaluation by a physician or licensed independent practitioner is conducted to determine the patient's current status, physical status, and any risks associated with the initiation or continuation of seclusion or restraint.[4]

Documentation regarding the decision to use seclusion should be objective and must support the need for such measures. Nurses are responsible to uphold these standards and to ensure that seclusion and restraints are not used as threats, as punishment, or for staff convenience. In the psychiatric setting, training focused on the prevention and use of seclusion and restraint must be provided during a staff member's orientation and at least annually thereafter.

### Right to Refuse Treatment

The right to refuse treatment often is regarded as a patient's right to refuse medication. Patients have the right to be provided sufficient information to make an informed decision about the risks and benefits of treatment, Patients have the right to refuse medications unless court ordered to take the medication or in emergent situations and then with limited use. Nurses are responsible for assessing and documenting objectively in such cases.

Nurses may believe that the benefits far outweigh the risks of psychiatric medication; however, patients retain the right to make this decision. In addition to concerns about side effects, there are a multitude of reasons why patients might refuse medications, including denial and lack of insight about mental illness, the cost of medications, and the stigma of taking a psychotropic medication.

Even patients who are under involuntary civil commitment and prisoners who are mentally ill do not forfeit all their civil liberties and have the right to refuse medication. There is a separate judicial process by which a patient can be determined to be incompetent to refuse medication, in which case medications may be court ordered.[6] Although psychiatric nurses can inform patients about benefits, risks, and alternatives to medication, forcing a patient to take medication, without the aforementioned exceptions, exposes nurses to possible liability.

### Confidentiality

Psychiatric nursing requires communication skills that promote trust and the sharing of personal information. The policy of confidentiality helps establish an environment of trust. Nurses must safeguard information shared by patients to be used for treatment purposes only except in cases otherwise required by law, such as reporting abuse or where release of information, such as for insurance purposes or continuity of care with other providers, has been granted.

The American Nurses Association Code of Ethics for Nurses,[7] many state nurse practice acts, and most agencies that treat the mentally ill have statements regarding patient confidentiality. Because of the nature of psychiatric care, patients must be able to trust that what is shared is used for their care and is not released to parties who have no need to know or no legal right to know.

Nurses protect confidentiality by discussing patient care matters in private areas and protecting the medical record by not leaving computer screens or documents accessible or within the view of others outside the treatment team; properly disposing of discarded documents, such as report sheets; and closing computer screens displaying patient information when not in use. Patient information sent by electronic methods, such as texting, must be done with encryption or with consent of the patient. When in doubt, proper consent for release of information should be obtained.

Everyone involved in a patient care is responsible for understanding and maintaining the regulations in regard to the HIPAA.[8] It is important for psychiatric nurses to understand that the rules that apply to psychiatric mental health practice are more stringent under HIPPA. The privacy of information relating to psychiatric mental health care and developmental disability services directly prohibits the disclosure of patient information relating to such services without written consent. The World Health Organization supports more stringent standards for patients with mental illness, stating, "Mental health legislation is necessary for protecting the rights of people with mental disorders, who are a vulnerable section of society. They face stigma, discrimination and marginalization in all societies, and this increases the likelihood that their human rights will be violated."[9]

Privileged communication is a right of patients that protects information from being shared with a court of law. Although lawyer-client and psychiatrist-patient privileged communication rules have been established, not all states clearly define privileged communication between nurse and patient.[10] There may be cases in which a nurse could be compelled to share in court information considered confidential. In some circumstances, breach of confidentiality is legal, including the duty to warn third parties under certain circumstances and mandated reporting of abuse, which are discussed subsequently.

### Duty to Protect

The principle—the duty to protect—states that when specific threats are made to a mental health provider about a specific victim, there is a duty to warn the intended victim. The Tarasoff decision from the 1970s[11] established a therapist's duty to protect third parties from foreseeable harm. In this case, a college student, Tatiana Tarasoff, was killed by a fellow student who had told his therapist of his plan to kill her and the therapist failed to inform the intended victim or her family.

There have been many variations among jurisdictions regarding the Tarasoff decision, which weigh a patient's right to confidentiality against the duty to protect a third party. In general, the duty to warn exists in cases when a patient makes a specific threat about a specific intended victim and in cases when a patient has a prior history of violence. Psychiatric nurses should be familiar with the laws pertaining to their jurisdiction. In general, clinicians are protected against breach of confidentiality when attempting in good faith to protect a third party.

### Mandated Reporting

Virtually all states have mandated reporting laws for nurses and other health care workers regarding suspected child and elder abuse and neglect. Some states have mandatory domestic violence reporting laws. State departments of social or human services oversee this reporting mechanism. There must be clear evidence of harm except in cases in which serious harm may result from neglect. Careful assessment and clinical judgment are invaluable in such cases.[12] Failure to follow reporting regulations is subject to legal action.

When reports are made with the intention of preventing harm, health care workers are protected from breach of confidentiality and civil action. Psychiatric home health nurses may find evidence of abuse or situations of imminent danger in patients' homes. In emergent situations, local law enforcement may be contacted. It may be helpful for home health nurses and other psychiatric nurses to inform patients of the duty to report during the initial assessment.[12]

## Informed Consent

Nurses are often involved in the process of assuring that a patient has willingly consented to treatment. Informed consent is not simply the signing of a form. Informed consent is the process by which information is shared about treatment options, risks, and alternatives. Nurses often are involved in this process, and it may involve written information and a patient being asked to sign a form. The patient must have the capacity to understand the proposed treatment, have adequate information to make a decision, not be coerced, and have the option to make a choice.[13]

## Treatment of Minors

Minors are considered legally incompetent to make treatment decisions for themselves, and parents of legal guardians have the right to make such decisions. The age of majority varies by state but is most often 18 years old. In general, persons younger than age 18 who are married or are in the military are considered emancipated minors. Some states also consider minors with children to be emancipated. Some jurisdictions make exceptions for minors to consent for certain types of treatment, such as substance abuse, prescribing contraceptives, treatment of sexually transmitted prevention, and suicide prevention.[14]

## Documentation

Documentation is the primary method by which the record of treatment, progress and response, and patient care are communicated. Additionally, for purposes of internal and external auditing, the medical record defines what occurred in treatment. In a court of law, the medical record defines what occurred in treatment. Documentation is an important nursing responsibility that must be thoughtful and complete.[15]

The most critical information in protection against a malpractice lawsuit is clinical documentation. Important clinical information should be documented in a clear factual statement. When documenting unusual actions or treatments, the rationale must be documented to support the course of treatment. Documentation is the first line of protection against legal liability. The use of electronic medical records where check boxes and cut-and-paste functions are offered can lead to incomplete charting of care. Many medical records today are electronic or have checklists that limit the possible responses. Although these methods often make nurses' work easier, they may be too restrictive to allow for complete and individualized documentation, and additional entries may be necessary.[16]

## Supervision and Safety

Nurses are key patient advocates essential to patient safety. The safety of patients with mental illness must be maintained in a variety of settings, such as the inpatient psychiatric setting and emergency department. Psychiatric nursing skills include awareness, sometimes referred to as intuition, of subtle changes that may signal concern. Nurses are called on to respond to changes in patient condition that may threaten patient safety.[17] Often, nonlicensed personnel provide and document monitoring of patients, yet the responsibility ultimately lies with the nurse to ensure that proper supervision occurs.

### Suicide Risk Assessment

One of the most crucial tasks of the psychiatric nurse is suicide risk assessment. As professionals who often have significant direct contact with patients, nurses play a key role in assessing the risk of suicide that may occur in a variety of settings, including outpatient clinics, inpatient psychiatric units, and emergency departments.[18] Although it is difficult to predict self-injurious behavior and it is rare for a nurse to be found liable in cases of completed suicide, thorough assessment and documentation are essential to decrease legal risk in cases of suicide.

Suicide risk assessment is a complex process that requires cooperation across disciplines and settings. Psychiatric nurses are often called on to provide expertise in this area. Training in suicide risk includes knowledge of screening tools, assessment skills optimizing the patient interview, prevention and intervention techniques, and the ability to apply this knowledge to clinical practice.[19]

## FORENSIC PSYCHIATRIC ISSUES (PERTAINING TO THE COURT SYSTEM)
### Civil Commitment Process

There were several factors that set in motion the mass exodus of patients from large state psychiatric hospitals a half century ago. Medicare and Medicaid, which are federal programs, were created in 1965, and patients living in state hospitals were not eligible for these benefits. As patients left the state hospitals, the cost of their care shifted from individual states to the federal government. The Lanterman-Petris-Short Act, also known as the California Community Mental Health Services Act of 1969, strictly limited the use of involuntary psychiatric admissions in duration and only in cases of imminent dangerousness. These standards implemented in California were soon replicated in other jurisdictions and are accepted standards of psychiatric care today, and the law currently favors individual freedoms of patients over societal concerns.[20,21]

Today, a wide variety of treatment settings exist, and inpatient treatment is reserved for patients who are mentally ill and require a high degree of monitoring for personal safety or the safety of others. Likewise, seclusion and restraint must be used only when other less restrictive means have been considered and ruled out.[20]

Civil commitment laws allow the state to treat a person with a mental illness without consent. Commitment laws are based on the "dangerousness standard" under which someone who is mentally ill can be involuntarily cared for when unable to care for himself or herself or when a danger to self or others. This process allows for family members or the police to seek commitment for persons with mental illness who are imminently dangerous yet refuse treatment.[21]

Specific criteria for commitment vary from one state to another. Common criteria for civil commitment include the stipulation that a person must have a mental illness, must lack the judgment to make decisions regarding hospitalization, and must be an immediate to harming self or others. Some states have statues pertaining specifically to alcohol and drug problems. Treatment is usually inpatient, although some jurisdictions allow outpatient civil commitment. Courts have ruled that nurses should not be found liable for holding a hospitalized patient who is later found wrongfully committed.[22]

Civil commitment laws of the past half century favor supporting civil liberties of the mentally ill, resulting in deinstitutionalization, have been blamed for increased homelessness, morbidity, and criminalization of the mentally ill.

## Competency

Within the criminal justice system, legal competency to stand trial is based on a defendant's ability to understand legal charges made and to aid an attorney in the defense. These criteria are referred to as the Dusky standard based on a 1960 Supreme Court case.[23] A person who lacks such capacity because of a severe mental illness or because of a severe developmental disability is considered legally incompetent. Defendants are considered competent unless there is some question about this presumption, usually raised by the person's behavior (eg, if the person exhibits bizarre behavior). Incompetence is not regarded as a static condition, and, if and when competence is reestablished, the person resumes the criminal process.

Other than competency to stand trial, there are many acts for which a patient might be considered competent within and outside the criminal justice system. For example, a patient agreeing to take medication or to undergo electroconvulsive therapy must be able to communicate a choice to be considered competent.

## Insanity Defense

The defense of insanity is used in the criminal process when a person is considered so severely mentally ill as to lack free choice or rationality at the time of committing an illegal act, that is, the person did not know right from wrong and did not make a conscious decision to commit the crime. Not all persons who are mentally ill meet the criteria for the insanity defense, and the criteria have some variation among jurisdictions. Persons found legally insane do not receive prison terms but typically are remanded to treatment in forensic hospitals. State laws vary regarding the criteria, disposition, and release from treatment regarding the insanity defense.[24]

The insanity defense has received a great deal of recent attention because of the 2002 trial of Andrea Yates. Yates was found guilty in the drowning deaths of her children despite unsuccessful arguments by her attorneys for a finding of innocence by reason of insanity. Yates had a long-standing history of depression and psychosis and was under the care of a psychiatrist. The prosecution did not dispute that Yates was mentally ill but argued that she knew it was wrong to drown her children yet made a decision to do so anyway.[25]

## LEGAL TRENDS
### Legal Issues in Advanced Practice

Advanced practice psychiatric nursing involves additional legal concerns. The scope of practice for the advanced practice registered nurse and requirements for the use of protocols, supervision, and other limitations vary widely from state to state and are outlined in each state's nursing practice act. The American Association of Nurse Practitioners is one of the largest national professional organizations, representing all advanced practice nurses. This organization provides valuable information, such as legislative and regulatory updates, evidence-based practice guidelines, and business management practice resources.[26] Many state nurses associations and other organizations have resources dedicated to advanced practice registered nurses.

Advanced practice registered nurses are exposed to liability through prescriptive authority, billing practice, and the unique nurse-patient relationship of therapy. There are 4 important elements of malpractice: duty of care, breach of the standard of care, injury, and injury caused by the breach of the standard of care. All advanced practice nurses should understand their scope of practice and duty of care. A breach in these important elements can place both patient and nurse at risk.[27,28]

A recent case involving both an advanced practice psychiatric-mental health nurse practitioner (PMHNP) and a family nurse practitioner (FNP) focused on medications prescribed by another clinician highlights the risk of liability. A patient was being treated by both an FNP and PMHNP in the same clinic. The FNP managed the patient's medication for hypertension. The PMHNP managed the patient's mental health medications, which consisted of lamotrigine. Shortly after the lamotrigine was initiated, the patient was assessed by the FNP with a complaint of body aches and the FNP prescribed an antibiotic. Four weeks later the patient followed up with the FNP for a rash, resulting in the addition of a steroid to treat the rash. The patient was hospitalized 2 days later with Stevens-Johnson syndrome and toxic epidermal necrolysis. The patient sued the FNP and clinic for damages incurred by a lengthy hospitalization. The FNP was found liable because she was responsible for recognizing side effects of all of the patient's medications, even those prescribed by others.[27,28]

### Liability Risks

Although there is no direct correlation to psychiatric nurses, it may be helpful to extrapolate data regarding malpractice claims against psychiatrists. For psychiatrists, the more severe a patient's illness, the higher the likelihood of legal action. Certification seems protective for psychiatrists, and psychiatric nurses should consider certification as validation of clinical expertise.

Common reasons for claims against psychiatrists include

- Incorrect treatment (often medications)
- Suicide or suicide attempt
- Confidentiality breach
- Drug interactions[29]

### Gun Laws and Mental Illness

An increase in the number of mass shootings in the United States, including the 2012 tragedy at Sandy Hook Elementary School, in which 20 children and 6 educators were killed, has fueled debates about gun regulations and the mentally ill. As far back as the Gun Control Act of 1968, which introduced mental health restrictions for gun sales, there has been an effort to restrict the purchasing of fire arms to those deemed a danger to themselves or others, by virtue of mental illness, who have been court mandated to treatment.[30]

The Brady Handgun Violence Prevention Act of 1993 required mandatory background checks for the purchase of weapons from federally licensed firearms dealers, restricting the sale of fire arms to the mentally ill who had been adjudicated to mental health care. The trading or purchasing of firearms from private individuals is more difficult to enforce. The National Instant Criminal Background Check System (NICS) allows for instant background checks; however, many states do not require mandatory reporting of mental health records into the system. Such was the case when in 2007 a young man who 2 years earlier had been court ordered to outpatient mental health care due to threat of danger to himself was able to pass an NICS background check to purchase weapons to use to kill students at Virginia Tech. Events at Virginia in

2007 Tech led to the federally passed NICS Improvement Amendments Act in 2008 designed in part to increase reporting of mental health records to the online system, yet states have been slow to respond to requirements to submit records, citing privacy concerns.[30]

It is difficult for trained professionals to predict violence and most persons with mental illness are not violent. Sadly, of the 31,000 annual deaths from shooting in the United States, a majority of those deaths are due to suicide. Approximately half of all suicides are committed with firearms, and death occurs 85% of the time when a gun is used. The debates regarding gun laws and mental illness will likely continue to rage.[30–32]

### Criminal Justice System and Mental Illness

As long-term psychiatric hospitals have closed and the number of inpatient psychiatric beds decrease, the numbers of prisons and jails with high populations of mentally ill have grown. Currently, approximately 3 times as many persons with mental illness are incarcerated as are in psychiatric hospitals. The psychiatric needs of prisoners are 4 times that of the general population. Poor access to mental health care may be a factor that contributes to persons with mental illness entering the criminal justice system.[33] Nurses who work with suspects, offenders, and victims of crimes are forensic psychiatric nurses, a specialty of growing need.[34]

### Mental Health Courts

In response to a disproportionate number of persons in the criminal justice system with mental health needs, there are a growing number of jurisdictions that utilize mental health courts for defendants with mental health disorders. The goal of mental health court is to divert persons charged with crimes away from incarceration and into treatment, thereby reducing criminal recidivism and improving mental health functioning. Individuals agree to court-monitored mental health treatment while avoiding jail time.[35,36]

### Disaster Nursing

The emergence of behavioral health services for world disasters is growing rapidly. World disasters, such as the 2015 bombings in Paris, France; terrorist acts of 9/11; and floods in India, are increasingly common. Mental health providers from around the world assist in responding to these disasters. The rules and regulations of the emergency operation system, such as the National Response Framework, apply to these situations as well as the local and national rules and regulations governing an industry. These emergencies are challenging in themselves but pose additional concerns. Special concern for psychiatric nurses are privacy issues, record keeping, relationships between provider and patient, and providing acute psychiatric services. What happens when legal rules and regulations governing a nurse in her home country conflict with another country in which services are provided? What is a nurse's legal liability and does immunity exist? These questions have yet to be clarified.[37]

### SUMMARY

The landscape of psychiatric nursing is rapidly changing. Psychiatric nurses are required to be well educated and knowledgeable with strong clinical skills, which are judged against standards acceptable of professional peers. Laws, agency policies, and regulations evolve over time as do clinical practice standards. In addition to basic education, psychiatric nurses must continually participate in professional development to understand changes in the field and develop new skills to meet these changes.[38,39] Becoming certified and involved in professional organizations is one way to help stay abreast of current trends and developments. To minimize the risk of litigation, nurses must be aware of laws, regulations, and standards that govern practice. Although it is critical for psychiatric nurses to practice with these parameters in mind, nothing can replace sound clinical judgment.

## REFERENCES

1. Joint Commission. Manual for joint commission national quality care. Available at: www.jointcommission.org/specifications_manual_joint_commission. Accessed November 30, 2015.
2. American Psychiatric Nurses Association, International Society of Psychiatric-Mental Health Nurses. Psychiatric-mental health nursing: Scope and standards of practice. (2nd edition). Silver Springs (MD): American Nurses Association; 2014.
3. Kane C. The 2014 scope and standards of practice for psychiatric mental health nursing: key updates. Online J Issues Nurs 2015;20(1):1.
4. Springer G. When and how to use restraints. Am Nurse Today 2015;10(1):26–7.
5. Federal register, December 8, 2006, 42 CFR, Part 482.
6. Wettstein RM. The right to refuse psychiatric treatment. Psychiatr Clin North Am 1999;22:173–82.
7. American Nurses Association. Code of ethics for nurses with interpretive statements. Washington, DC: American Nurses Association; 2015.
8. U.S. Department of Health & Human Services. The Health Insurance Portability and Accountability Act of 1996 (HIPAA) Privacy, Security and Breach Notification Rules. 2015. Available at: http://www.hhs.gov/ocr/privacy/. Accessed November 30, 2015.
9. World Health Organziation. Mental health legislation & human rights. 2015. Available at: http://www.who.int/mental_health/resources/en/Legislation.pdf. Accessed November 30, 2015.
10. Wysoker A. Confidentiality. J Am Psychiatr Nurses Assoc 2001;7:57–8.
11. Vitaly Tarasoff et al. plantiffs and appellants v the regents of the University, et al. defendants and respondent, SF 23042. (1976). Pacific Reporter, 551p.2d, 334–62.
12. Dubowitz H, Giardiano A, Gustavson E. Child neglect: guidelines for pediatricians. Pediatr Rev 2000;21:111–6.
13. Schouten R. Law and psychiatry: what should our residents learn? Harv Rev Psychiatry 2001;9:36–8.
14. Muscari ME. When can an adolescent give consent. Am J Nurs 1998;98:18–9.
15. Mohr WK. Deconstructing the language of psychiatric hospitalization. J Adv Nurs 1999;79:1052–9.
16. Knoll JL. The psychiatrist's duty to protect. CNS Spectr 2015;20(03):215–22.
17. Dresser S. The role of nursing surveillance in keeping patients safe. J Nurs Adm 2012;42(7–8):361–8.
18. Good B, Walsh RM, Alexander G. Assessment of the acute psychiatric patient in the emergency department: legal cases and caveats. West J Emerg Med 2014; 15(3):312–7.
19. Grant CL, Lusk JL. A multidisciplinary approach to therapeutic risk management of the suicidal patient. J Multidiscip Healthc 2015;8:291–8.

20. Torrey EF. The insanity offense: how America's failure to treat the seriously mentally ill endangers its citizens. New York: WW Morton and Company; 2008.
21. Slovenko R. Criminal law standards in civil commitment. J Psychiatry Law 2012; 40:135–45.
22. Large MM, Neilssen OB, Lackersteen SM. Did the introduction of 'dangerousness' and 'risk of harm' criteria in mental health laws increase the incidence of suicide in the United States? Soc Psychiatry Psychiatr Epidemiol 2009;44: 614–21.
23. Gendel MH. Forensic and medical legal issues in addiction psychiatry. Psychiatr Clin North Am 2004;27:611–26.
24. Dusky v US, 363 US 402 (1960).
25. Torry ZD, Weiss K. Medication noncompliance and criminal responsibility: is the insanity defense legitimate? J Psychiatry Law 2012;40(2):219–42.
26. Asher E, Markley M. Victim's right's group praises verdict, yates backers:mental illness misunderstood. Houston (TX): Houston Chronicle; 2002. p. 29.
27. American Association of Nurse Practitioners (AANP). 2015. Available at: https://www.aanp.org/about-aanp. Accessed November 30, 2015.
28. Buppert C. The nurse practitioner's business practice and legal guide. Sudbury (MA): Jones & Bartlett Publishers; 2014. Available at: www.jblearning.com.
29. NSO, NP 2012 Liability. Available at: www.nso.com. Accessed November 30, 2015.
30. Reich J, Schatzberg A. An empirical data comparison of regulatory agency and malpractice legal problems for psychiatrist. Ann Clin Psychiatry 2014;26(2):91–6.
31. Goss KA. Defying the odds on gun regulation: the passage of bipartisan mental health laws across the states. Am J Orthopsychiatry 2015;85(3):203–10.
32. Swanson JW. Mental illness and new gun law reforms. JAMA 2013;309:1233–4.
33. Applebaum PS. "One madman keeping loaded guns" Misconceptions of mental illness and their legal consequences. Psychiatr Serv 2004;55(10):1105–6.
34. Kanapaux W. Guilty of mental illness. Psych Times 2004;21(1):40–50.
35. Brown KM. From nurse Ratched to modern forensic mental health nursing. J Psychiatry Law 2012;40:93–104.
36. Honegger LN. Does the evidence support the case for mental health courts? A review of the literature. Law Hum Behav 2015;39(5):478–88.
37. Burke MM, Griggs M, Dykens EM, et al. Defendants with intellectual disabilities and mental health diagnoses: faring in a mental health court. J Intellect Disabil Res 2012;56(3):305–16.
38. Flynn BW, Speier AH. Disaster behavioral health: legal and ethical considerations in a rapidly changing field. Curr Psychiatry Rep 2014;16(8):1–8.
39. Kesselheim AS, Studdert DM. The supreme court, preemption, and malpractice liability. N Engl J Med 2009;360(6):559–61.

# Caring for the Patient with an Anxiety Disorder

Deborah Antai-Otong, MS, APRN, PMHCNS-BC, FAAN

## KEYWORDS

- Anxiety disorders • Cognitive-behavioral theory • Cognitive processing therapy
- Antidepressants • Co-occurring disorders • Person-centered care

## KEY POINTS

- Anxiety disorders are prevalent, costly, and potentially debilitating.
- Anxiety disorders have a co-occurrence with depression, substance use disorders, and medical disorders.
- Anxiety disorders have complex neurobiological underpinnings mediated by environmental, genetic, social, and cultural factors.
- Anxiety disorders are the most common reason that patients seek psychiatric and medical services in primary care settings.
- Nurses are poised to identify patients experiencing anxiety disorders and evidence-based treatment options.

Anxiety disorders are among the most widespread of mental health conditions, and may be recurring or chronic, with an estimated lifetime prevalence of more than 15%.[1] Research further indicates that the incidence of anxiety disorder wanes in older adults and that it is commonly found in women.[2] These disorders are primary reasons that people seek medical and psychiatric treatment and are often a precursor to co-existing mood disorders.[3] Anxiety disorders cause a considerable burden of distress and functional disability similar to other medical conditions, such as diabetes and cancer.[4,5]

Anxiety disorders have a predictable debilitating course of anxiety and reduced productivity and interference with functioning and quality of life. Findings from a 12-month study conducted by Kessler and his colleagues[6] of the lifetime prevalence and morbidity risk of anxiety and mood disorders indicate that the prevalence of anxiety disorders varies with age of onset.[7] The most common early onset anxiety disorders include specific phobias, social anxiety disorder (SAD) or social phobia, and

---

This article is an update of an article previously published in Nursing Clinics of North America, Volume 38, Issue 1, March 2003.
Disclosure: None.
Department of Veterans Affairs, Veterans Integrated Service Networks-(VISN-17), 2301 E. Lamar Boulevard, Arlington, TX 76006, USA
*E-mail address:* Deborah.Antai-Otong@va.gov

Nurs Clin N Am 51 (2016) 173–183
http://dx.doi.org/10.1016/j.cnur.2016.01.003
0029-6465/16/$ – see front matter © 2016 Elsevier Inc. All rights reserved.

separation anxiety. Generalized anxiety disorder and panic disorder tend to occur most often in mid to later life.[6] These disorders are most likely to co-exist with medical conditions and other psychiatric or substance use disorders.

## ECONOMIC AND PERSONAL COSTS OF ANXIETY DISORDERS

The cost of anxiety disorders is large because of the financial and personal toll they have on individuals and society. The cost of these disorders may be mitigated with increased health education, early detection, and person-centered interventions. In 2010, the World Economic Forum reported that the results of a 20-year project involving the cost of several chronic medical conditions, including mental health, yielded an estimated cumulative loss of productivity of about $47 trillion dollars, which is about 75% of the world gross domestic product.[4,5,8] Estimates from this report further show that the global cost involving psychiatric disorders, including anxiety disorders, was $2.5 trillion with a projected cost increase of $6 trillion in 2030. There is a general consensus that anxiety and other psychiatric disorders increase the risk, worsen the course, increase health care use, and worsen treatment outcomes for medical conditions such as diabetes and cardiovascular events.[4,5,8] Data from a 12-month study showed that posttraumatic stress disorder (PTSD) and panic disorder contribute to the highest rates of heath care use. These data also indicate that all anxiety disorders reduced workplace performance and significantly interfered with quality of life. Patients with anxiety disorders are more likely to seek treatment, complaining of co-existing disorders, especially depression, with a history of early onset and more severe symptoms than patients with a single disorder.[3,4,9] Anxiety disorders interfere significantly with overall functioning because of distress that is sometimes more agonizing than physical pain. In addition, depending on the type of anxiety disorder, patients may report acute panic and recurrent tormenting intrusive thoughts or images, think that they are dying or going crazy, or experience unbearable and immobilizing obsessions and associated behavioral disturbances.[10] For these reasons, nurses and other health care providers are challenged to identify symptoms of diverse anxiety disorders and co-existing conditions, such as depression and substance use disorders, and initiate evidence-based interventions.

New treatment initiatives have advanced improvements in the understanding and treatment of anxiety disorders. Understanding anxiety disorders requires a brief overview of complex causes and treatment implications. This article discusses several anxiety disorders and treatment planning: panic disorder, generalized anxiety disorder (GAD), SAD, PTSD, and obsessive compulsive disorder (OCD).

## CAUSES OF ANXIETY DISORDERS

Most research indicates that anxiety disorders are complex and arise from intricate neurochemical, neuroanatomic, neuroinflammatory, genetic, neuroendocrinologic, and psychoimmunologic factors.[11,12] Cognitive-behavioral and environmental and stress factors also play a role in anxiety disorders.

Neurochemical theories indicate dysregulation of a host of neurotransmitters, including excitatory neurotransmitters, such as noradrenalin and glutamate; and inhibitory neurotransmitters, such as gamma-aminobutyric acid and serotonin. Additional data indicate neurochemistry alterations in dopamine metabolites in cerebral spinal fluid, reduced sensitivity in postsynaptic dopamine, and dysregulation in endogenous opioid systems. Support of the neurochemistry theory is seen in the efficacy of pharmacologic agents, such as benzodiazepines for acute anxiety and various antidepressants, including serotonin reuptake inhibitors (eg, sertraline, fluoxetine), and serotonin-norepinephrine reuptake inhibitors (eg, venlafaxine).[13] There is further evidence that supports the use cognitive enhancers, such as D-cycloserine and yohimbine in the regulation and treatment of contextual information in fear extinction, specifically the acquisition, consolidation, and retrieval of fear-based memories.[14]

Neuroanatomic alterations include imprinting or memory consolidation of emotionally traumatic memories and conditioned fear that are mediated through dopamine 1 and dopamine 2 receptor signaling in the amygdala through the posterior hippocampus and avoidance conditioning mediated through the ventromedial prefrontal cortex.[14,15]

Psychoimmunologic or immune-mediated theories suggest that various anxiety disorders, particularly PTSD and OCD, may compromise the immune system. These theories arise from the studies that indicate that alterations in the hypothalamic-pituitary-adrenal axis and increased levels of the glucocorticoid hormone cortisol and proinflammatory and antiinflammatory cytokines contribute to the neurogenesis of various anxiety disorders. The precise basis of these assumptions is unclear, but prevailing findings show that individuals with PTSD and other anxiety disorders are more likely to have medical conditions associated with prolonged immunosuppression, such as rheumatoid arthritis, irritable bowel syndrome, and cardiovascular disease.[16,17]

Genetic predisposition contributes to anxiety disorders. Family aggregated and twin studies support the role of genetic influence and heritability of various anxiety disorders, such as OCD.

Cognitive-behavioral theorists assert that anxious individuals often hold irrational or distorted beliefs about themselves, others, and the future. They tend to overgeneralize or exaggerate a potential for catastrophic situations and negative consequences (eg, "My son failed his class, thus, I must be a bad mother" or "If I assert myself, people will not like me").[18] Environmental factors and stress issues also contribute to anxiety disorders, particularly acute stress or PTSD, which are associated with an overwhelming traumatic or life-threatening situation or exposure.

## SPECIFIC ANXIETY DISORDERS
### Panic Disorder

Panic disorder is a common anxiety disorder characterized by discrete or unexpected, unprovoked periods of intense fear or dread (cognitive); physical distress (biological), avoidance (behavioral), or all three. It affects 2% to 3% of the general population.[6,10] Chief complaints of panic disorder[9] include the following:

- Increased heart rate, blood pressure, and respiration rate
- Palpitations
- Diaphoresis (sweating)
- Shortness of breath
- Dizziness
- Derealization (environment feels unreal) or depersonalization (out-of-body experience)
- Tremulousness or shakiness
- Gastrointestinal distress ("butterflies," nausea, diarrhea)
- Numbness or tingling sensations (paresthesias)
- Hot flashes or chills
- Chest pain or discomfort
- Fear of dying, going crazy, or being out of control

### Agoraphobia

Panic disorder may exist with or without agoraphobia and agoraphobia may exist without panic disorder. The prevalence of agoraphobia among adults is 1.7%.[6] Agoraphobia characteristically includes intense fear or anxiety involving 2 or more of the following situations:

- Traveling on public transportation (eg, automobiles, subways)
- Being in open spaces (eg, shopping malls)
- Being in closed and crowded places (eg, theaters, elevators)
- Being outside of the home alone
- Places with limited escape routes (these are actively avoided)[10]

The frequency of panic attacks varies. However, characteristically, patients have 2 or 4 attacks per week and complain of a sudden, rapid onset of symptoms that peak in 10 minutes and abate within 60 minutes. Patients may report anticipatory anxiety with 1 or more phobias arising from environmental stimuli, such as open spaces, crowds, or highways. At least 4 of the symptoms listed earlier must be present during at least 1 of the panic episodes or attacks. Panic disorder produces significant distress, and patients tend to have marked social impairment that interferes with their level of functioning. Because patients with Panic disorder tend to have co-existing conditions, such as depression and substance use disorder, these conditions must be ruled out and treated with appropriate interventions.[9] Physical symptoms of panic attacks can also mimic serious medical conditions, such as a heart attack or seizure, and, similar to psychiatric conditions, they must be ruled out and treated accordingly. Nurses play a key role in assessing and treating patients with various anxiety disorders. This process begins by establishing rapport and allaying distress by reassuring and explaining all procedures. Asking how long the patient has had the symptoms and what has been helpful in the past, as well as additional questions concerning the medications they are taking and when they last had a physical examination, are helpful in establishing a differential diagnosis. The biopsychosocial assessment provides information about symptoms and duration; sociocultural factors and context; past treatment; dietary intake, including caffeine use, beverages, and over-the-counter preparations; sleeping patterns; and present stressors. In addition, taking vital signs; performing a mental status examination that includes questions about suicide risk, including current and past thoughts of suicide; and ordering or reviewing the results of diagnostic tests, such as electrocardiograms and blood work, provide valuable information. Patients are often reassured and relieved when they are told their results are normal and they are not dying or going crazy. When an accurate diagnosis is established, appropriate treatment can be initiated.

### Treatment Considerations

Before initiating any treatment of anxiety disorders, the patient must have a complete and thorough physical examination and mental status examination. These examinations are necessary to rule out other medical and psychiatric conditions, such as metabolic disorders or syndromes, including diabetes and thyroid disease; cardiovascular disease; and substance use disorders, including those associated with central nervous system stimulants and alcohol withdrawal. When a differential diagnosis is made, treatment can be initiated.

Mainstay treatment of patients with panic disorder, with or without agoraphobia, should target several areas and include pharmacologic and nonpharmacologic interventions. The biological symptoms can be managed with pharmacologic interventions, such as benzodiazepines (eg, clonazepam) for acute anxiety and antidepressants (eg, paroxetine, escitalopram) to reduce the frequency of attacks and severity of symptoms. Nonpharmacologic interventions include cognitive behavior therapy and stress management techniques, including progressive muscle relaxation, abdominal deep breathing exercises, and visualization.

Other treatment considerations are as follows:

### Provide health education
This intervention is crucial because it provides patients and families with important information about causative factors, symptoms, evidence-based interventions, and health promoting and maintenance activities, such as mindfulness meditation and stress and anger management techniques. Health education is empowering and reassuring to patients and families concerning symptom management, treatment options, and quality of life. Health education can be offered in various venues, including offices, online chat or discussion groups, emails, and instant messaging.

### Minimize avoidant behaviors
Exposure and cognitive behavior therapies assist patients in desensitization of stressful situations, such as highways and open spaces. Pharmacologic interventions offer the biological relief and reduction of symptoms that is necessary to improve cognitive functioning. Exposure therapy is a behavioral technique that involves exposing the patient to a feared object or situation (eg, open spaces, such as a mall or highway) within a safe and nonthreatening setting to help reduce the fear-provoked anxiety. Exposure therapy sessions lasting 2 hours or more are more effective than sessions lasting 1 hour. During this intervention, the patients are asked to imagine their worst anxiety-provoking situations for 20 minutes before using cognitive restructuring (challenging distortions as exaggerations or overestimation). During these sessions, the patients acquire health information that challenges irrational or distorted cognitions or beliefs about the event or situations.[19–21]

### Challenge distorted cognitions (same as suppressing avoidant behaviors)
Cognitive behavior therapy also involves using homework assignments to enable patients to keep logs or diaries and self-monitor anxiety-provoking situations, and provides ways to challenge distorted cognitions.[19–21] Cognitive behavior therapy is an active, problem-solving approach that teaches patients adaptive coping strategies to alleviate symptoms and distress. This approach also involves using relaxation techniques to reduce biological arousal.

### Provide long-term monitoring
Long-term monitoring is provided to prevent relapse (pharmacologic and nonpharmacologic interventions) to reduce distressful and sometimes overwhelming symptoms and relapse and to facilitate a high level of functioning and improve quality of life.

### Assess for coexisting disorders, such as depression and substance use disorders
When coexisting conditions exist, appropriate treatment should be initiated. In the case of depression, which is highly prevalent in patients with panic disorder, antidepressants are appropriate. In the case of a substance use disorder (history or active), benzodiazepines should be avoided except in the case of alcohol withdrawal. Buspirone is more appropriate for these patients; it is not appropriate for acute anxiety, but is helpful in treating long-term anxiety without the risk of dependence, abuse, or relapse. Because of the prevalence and coexistence of depression,[1–3] these patients must be assessed continuously for suicide and other high-risk behaviors.

*Use technologies to increase access*
Therapy-supported Internet-based CBT,[21] telemental health, online discussion groups or chat rooms, and media-based treatment should be considered as alternative treatment modalities. In some cases, these approaches have similar clinical outcomes to face-to-face services in this patient population.[22–24] Considerations to use technologies, such as the Internet, chat rooms, and online group discussions, require strict adherence to policies and procedures related to information security, privacy, confidentiality, and informed consent.

### Generalized Anxiety Disorder

GAD is a prevalent psychiatric disorder that affects about 2.9% of adults and 0.9% of adolescents.[6] Similar to other anxiety disorders, GAD carries a substantial risk of disability and poor quality of life. GAD tends to have an early onset with duration of more than 5 years.

The chronicity and longitudinal course of anxiety disorders, including GAD, is influenced by partner status; age of onset; history of childhood trauma; coexisting psychiatric disorders, including depression and bipolar disorder; and substance use disorders.[24,25] Research indicates that a high co-occurrence of these disorders is characteristic of the course and nature of GAD and is associated with significant disability, interference with function, and reduced quality of life. The co-existence of these disorders has important clinical implications for its course and treatment outcomes.[25] GAD is costly and prevalent in primary care settings. It is one of the most common diagnoses in patients with unexplained physical symptoms.[26] Implications for nurses include identification of symptoms; health education; assessment of co-existing conditions, such as mood and substance use disorders; and risk of danger to self and others.

An essential feature of GAD is excessive worrying occurring more days than not for at least 6 months. Patients also experience an array of physical symptoms, such as feeling keyed up and sleep disturbances. In addition, the diagnosis of GAD involves at least 3 of the following[10]:

- Fatigue
- Restlessness
- Impaired concentration
- Irritability
- Muscle tension
- Sleep disturbances
- Gastrointestinal distress
- Feeling keyed up or edgy[10]

### Treatment Considerations

As previously mentioned, patients with anxiety disorders must have a complete physical examination and mental status examination to make a differential diagnosis. When a differential diagnosis of GAD is confirmed, pharmacologic and nonpharmacologic interventions can be initiated. Because GAD is a chronic and recurring psychiatric disorder, the patients require long-term treatment to prevent relapse.

Pharmacologic interventions for GAD include antidepressants, such as selective serotonin reuptake inhibitors (SSRIs) and serotonin norepinephrine reuptake inhibitors (SNRIs). These drugs also are beneficial for patients with co-existing mood disorders.[27,28] Nonpharmacologic interventions are the same as those used to treat panic disorder and include cognitive behavior therapy, including Internet and online services; relaxation techniques; mindfulness meditation; and stress management. Nurses can develop person-centered care planning by encouraging patients to identify their strengths, preferences, and abilities to develop hobbies, and focus on areas in which they have control. Providing structure and opportunities to succeed increases the patients' self-esteem and self-efficacy. Family involvement is also crucial to successful treatment outcomes. Providing health education and referrals to community family support groups, Internet chat rooms, and online discussions may allay family members' anxiety and promote understanding of their loved ones' conditions. Because of the high incidence of mood disorders, including depression and substance use disorders, these patients must be assessed continuously for their level of dangerousness toward themselves and others.

### Social Anxiety Disorder (Social Phobia)

Similar to other anxiety disorders, SAD is chronic psychiatric disorder, with a lifetime prevalence of 7%.[6] SAD produces significant interference with function, personally and professionally. Likewise, SAD often coexists with other psychiatric disorders, such as depression and substance use disorder.[1,3,5,7] The onset of social phobia occurs during adolescence, with a median age of 13 years, when interpersonal relationships are significant, and plays a role in adult relationships. Clinical features of SAD arise from exposure to feared social situations and production of marked and persistent fear and intense anxiety caused by 1 or more social performance situations, scrutiny by others, and avoidant behaviors.[10]

### Treatment Considerations

When a differential diagnosis has been made and SAD is confirmed, pharmacologic interventions include short-term benzodiazepines (eg, clonazepam) and antidepressant agents (SSRIs, SNRIs).[20,29] Nonpharmacologic interventions are similar to those used to treat those patients with panic disorder and GAD and include monitoring the patient for relapse and risk of dangerousness to self and others. Nurses play pivotal roles in helping patients and their families understand and cope with this disorder. Role rehearsal or role playing are excellent tools that promote a sense of competence and confidence in dealing with anxiety-provoking events. Teaching assertiveness training and relaxation techniques along with conflict resolution offers patients an opportunity to deal with stressful situations effectively.

### Posttraumatic Stress Disorder

The lifetime prevalence of PTSD in the United States is high at about 8%, with a higher incidence among Veterans and inner city populations.[6,7] There is a higher prevalence of PTSD among women, previously married individuals, military service personnel, combat veterans,[30,31] and individuals who experience various traumas (eg, child abuse, intimate partner violence, rape).[10] PTSD is characterized by responses to an overwhelming and traumatic event that emerge 1 month after exposure to trauma, with 4 sets of symptoms, which are listed in **Box 1**.

### Treatment Considerations

When a diagnosis of PTSD has been confirmed, treatment must center on the patient's presenting symptoms and reduction of the chronic course. Similar to other psychiatric disorders, PTSD coexists with depression, substance use disorders, other anxiety disorders, and medical conditions, including traumatic brain injury, chronic pain, and sleep disorders. A thorough history of the event, emergence of symptoms, and duration is crucial to making an accurate diagnosis of PTSD and initiating evidence-based

---

**Box 1**
**PTSD symptoms**

1. Intrusive symptoms
   A. Intrusive and distressful images or thoughts of event
   B. Flashbacks
   C. Nightmares and sleep disturbances

2. Avoidance behaviors
   A. Avoidance of the situation or reminders of the event
   B. Numbness
   C. Psychological amnesias

3. Negative cognitions and mood associated with the trauma
   A. Startle response
   B. Hypervigilance
   C. Concentration disturbances
   D. Negative emotional states (eg, fear, guilt, sadness, shame)
   E. Loss of awareness of present surroundings (derealization)
   F. Numbness
   G. Psychological amnesias

4. Intense alterations in arousal and reactivity
   A. Irritable behavior and angry outbursts with little provocation (eg, aggressive behaviors);
      hypervigilance
   B. Exaggerated startle or stress response
   C. Sleep disturbances[10]

---

treatment planning. Each patient handles trauma individually. Nurses must use a strength-based approach and use trauma-informed care in the treatment of PTSD. Use the patient's verbal and nonverbal cues to guide the assessment process and avoid pressing for a description of trauma to prevent retraumatizing.

Pharmacologic interventions for PTSD include antidepressant medications, such as SSRIs and SNRIs.[19,29] Nonpharmacologic interventions include cognitive behavior therapies, such as cognitive processing therapy and prolonged exposure therapy,[30] and anger management. Group therapy and other support groups are helpful for patients and for family members. Psychotherapies provided through various technologies, including the Internet, tele–mental health technologies (eg, clinical video teleconferencing, mobile devices), and online group discussions and chat rooms offer additional venues to receive services. An in-depth discussion of PTSD is provided in the article (see Deborah Antai-Otong: Caring for trauma survivors, in this issue).

Similar to other anxiety disorders, PTSD places a large burden on families. Nurses must assess the patient and family needs and educate them about pharmacologic and nonpharmacologic symptom management, such as marital and family therapy. Nurses must also assess the risk of dangerousness to self and others and monitor for signs of substance use disorders.

### Obsessive Compulsive Disorder

Patients with OCD often complain of persistent, intrusive thoughts and images (obsessions) and the urge to perform repetitive and ritualistic behaviors (compulsions). The patients recognize that these thoughts and rituals are unrealistic and irrational, but feel that they have no control over them. Similar to other anxiety disorders, OCD is a chronic psychiatric disorder with an unremitting course. The prevalence of OCD is approximately 1.2% and men and women are equally likely to be affected. OCD is potentially debilitating and the degree of functional distress often parallels the nature of the obsessions and rituals and the management of symptoms. OCD has been recategorized in the Diagnostic and Statistical Manual of Mental Disorders, Fifth Edition, as a separate category and renamed as OCD and related disorders, which includes body dysmorphic disorder, hoarding, trichotillomania, and excoriation (skin picking).[10] This article focuses on OCD as it relates to anxiety. Similar to other anxiety disorders, OCD has a high coexistence with depression and substance use disorders.[10]

Characteristic symptoms of OCD are obsessions and compulsions. If patients are obsessed about cleanliness, after shaking hands with someone they might have intrusive thoughts of contamination (obsessions) from the hand shake and be driven to wash their hands repeatedly to remove germs (compulsions). The intrusive thoughts generate intense anxiety, biological symptoms, and concentration disturbances that are relieved only by excessive handwashing (ritualistic behavior).[10]

### Treatment Considerations

Treatment must begin with a complete physical examination and mental status examination to make a definitive diagnosis. Pharmacologic interventions include antidepressants, such as SSRIs (fluvoxamine) and tricyclic antidepressants (eg, clomipramine).[20,29] Relapse rates are high when these medications are discontinued, suggesting that long-term maintenance treatment is necessary to improve symptom management and ultimately the patients' quality of life and functional status. Nonpharmacologic interventions include those that were previously discussed for other anxiety disorders, such as assessing the patient's level of dangerousness to self and others and signs of substance use disorder. Educating patients and families about treatment options and symptoms to report is crucial to successful treatment planning.

## SUMMARY

Anxiety disorders are among the most prevalent and disabling psychiatric conditions. Patients now have a plethora of treatment options and venues to manage these potentially disabling and costly psychiatric conditions. Anxiety disorders represent a large portion of primary care visits in diverse practice settings. Nurses are in key positions to identify symptoms of various anxiety disorders, initiate appropriate treatment, and make appropriate referrals. Families play a key role in successful treatment planning and must be an integral part of the health care team. Major nursing interventions must focus on understanding the underpinnings of anxiety disorders as target sites for pharmacologic and nonpharmacologic interventions, on collaborating with patients, family members, and other providers, and on initiating evidence-based treatment to patients presenting with anxiety disorders.

## REFERENCES

1. Kessler RC, Aguilar-Gaxiola S, Alonso J, et al. The global burden of mental disorders: an update from the WHO World Mental Health (WMH) surveys. Epidemiol Psichiatr Soc 2009;18(1):23–33.

2. Byers AI, Yaffee K, Covinsky KE, et al. High occurrence of mood and anxiety disorders among older adults: the National Comorbidity Survey Replication. Arch Gen Psychiatry 2010;67:489–96.

3. Bener A, Abou-Saleh MT, Dafeeah EE, et al. The prevalence and burden of psychiatric disorders in primary health care visits in Qatar: too little time? J Family Med Prim Care 2015;4:89–95.

4. Wittchen HU, Jacobi F, Rehm J, et al. The size and burden of mental disorders and other disorders of the brain in Europe 2010. Eur Neuropsychopharmacol 2011;21:655–79.
5. Whiteford HA, Degenhardt L, Rehm J, et al. Global burden of disease attributable to mental and substance use disorders: findings from the Global Burden of Disease Study 2010. Lancet 2013;382:1575–86.
6. Kessler RC, Petulhova M, Sampson NA, et al. Twelve-month and lifetime prevalence and lifetime morbid risk of anxiety and mood disorders in the United States. Int J Methods Psychiatr Res 2012;21:169–84.
7. Breslau N, Peterson EL, Schultz LR. A second look at prior trauma and the posttraumatic stress disorder effects of subsequent trauma: a prospective epidemiological study. Arch Gen Psychiatry 2008;65:431–7.
8. Bloom DE, Cafiero ET, Jané-Llopis E, et al. The global economic burden of noncommunicable diseases. Geneva (Switzerland): World Economic Forum; 2011.
9. Ho AK, Thorpe CT, Pandhi N, et al. Association of anxiety and depression with hypertension control: a US multidisciplinary group practice observational study. J Hypertens 2015;33:2215–22.
10. American Psychiatric Association. Diagnostic and statistical manual of mental disorders. 5th edition. Washington, DC: Author; 2013.
11. Furtad M, Katzman MA. Neuroinflammatory pathways in anxiety, posttraumatic stress, and obsessive compulsive disorders. Psychiatry Res 2015;229:37–48.
12. Meir DS, Merz CJ, Hamacher-Dang TC, et al. Effects of cortisol on reconsolidation of reactivated fear memories. Neuropsychopharmacology 2015;40:3036–43.
13. Mayo-Wilson E, Dias S, Mavranezouli I, et al. Psychological and pharmacological interventions for social anxiety disorder in adults: a systematic review and network meta-analysis. Lancet Psychiatry 2014;1:368–76.
14. Singewaldk N, Schmuckermair C, Whittle N, et al. Pharmacology of cognitive enhancers for exposure-based therapy of fear, anxiety and trauma-related disorders. Pharmacol Ther 2015;149:150–90.
15. Haaker J, Lonsdorf TB, Kalisch R. Effects of post-extinction L-DOPA administration on the spontaneous recovery and reinstatement of fear in a human fMRI study. Eur Neuropsychopharmacol 2015;25:1544–55.
16. Griffin GD, Charron D, Al-Daccak R. Post-traumatic stress disorder: revisiting adrenergics, glucocorticoids, immune system effects and homeostasis. Clin Transl Immunology 2014;3:e27.
17. Jergovic M, Bendelja K, Savic Mlakar A, et al. Circulating levels of hormones, lipids, and immune mediators in post-traumatic stress disorder - a 3-month follow-up study. Front Psychiatry 2015;14(6):49.
18. Bergin J, Verhulst B, Aggen SH, et al. Obsessive compulsive symptom dimensions and neuroticism: an examination of shared genetic and environmental risk. Am J Med Genet B Neuropsychiatr Genet 2014;165B:647–53.
19. Beck AT, Emery G, Greenberg R. Anxiety disorder and phobias: a cognitive perspective. New York: Basic Books; 1985.
20. Bandelow B, Zohar J, Hollander E, et al, WFSBP Task Force on treatment guidelines for anxiety, obsessive-compulsive and post-traumatic stress disorders. World Federation of Societies of Biological Psychiatry (WFSBP) guidelines for the pharmacological treatment of anxiety, obsessive-compulsive and posttraumatic stress disorders – first revision. World J Biol Psychiatry 2008;9:248–312.
21. Abramowitz JS, Deacon BJ, Whiteside SPH. Exposure therapy for anxiety: principles and practice. New York: Guilford Press; 2010.

22. Sars D, van Minnen A. On the use of exposure therapy in the treatment of anxiety disorders: a survey among cognitive behavioural therapists in the Netherlands. BMC Psychol 2015;3:26, eCollection 2015.
23. Olthius JV, Watt MC, Bailey K, et al. Therapist-supported Internet cognitive behavioural therapy for anxiety disorders in adults. Cochrane Database Syst Rev 2015;(3):CD011565.
24. Backhaus A, Agha Z, Maglione ML, et al. Videoconferencing psychotherapy: a systematic review. Psychol Serv 2012;2012(9):111–31.
25. Batelaan NM, Rhebergen D, Spinhoven P, et al. Two-year course trajectories of anxiety disorders: do DSM classifications matter? J Clin Psychiatry 2014;75:985–93.
26. Schaffer A, McIntosh D, Goldstein BI, et al. The CANMAT task force recommendations for the management of patients with mood disorders and comorbid anxiety disorders. Ann Clin Psychiatry 2012;24:6–22.
27. Alosaimi FD, Al-Sultan O, Alghamdi Q, et al. Association of help-seeking behavior with depression and anxiety disorders among gastroenterological patients in Saudi Arabia. Saudi J Gastroenterol 2014;20:233–40.
28. Levitan MN, Papelbaum N, Nardi AE. Profile of agomelatine and its potential in the treatment of generalized anxiety disorder. Neuropsychiatr Dis Treat 2015;5:1149–55.
29. Bandelow B, Reitt M, Rover C, et al. Efficacy of treatments for anxiety disorders: a meta-analysis. Int Clin Psychopharmacol 2015;30:183–92.
30. Bernardy NC, Friedman MJ. Psychopharmacological strategies in the management of posttraumatic stress disorder (PTSD): what have we learned? Curr Psychiatry Rep 2015;17:564.
31. Steenkamp MM, Litz BT, Hoge CW, et al. Psychotherapy for military-related PTSD: a review of randomized clinical trials. JAMA 2015;314:489–500.

# Assessing and Treating the Patient with Acute Psychotic Disorders

Lisa Jensen, DNP, APRN, PMHCNS-BC[a],*,
Rebecca Clough, MSN, APRN, PMHCNS-BC[b]

## KEYWORDS

- Acute psychosis • Schizophrenia • Verbal de-escalation • Therapeutic alliance
- Pharmacologic interventions • Movement disorders

## KEY POINTS

- Patients with acute psychosis may present to the ED with agitation.
- Safety is paramount in these situations.
- Accurate assessment is important to ensure appropriate treatment.
- Nurses are involved in the assessment and the de-escalation of patients with acute psychosis.

## INTRODUCTION

Emergency departments (ED) frequently are faced with managing agitated patients experiencing episodes of acute psychosis. These situations can escalate quickly into a crisis, resulting in frustration for the staff members and a dangerous environment for patients, visitors, and staff. Effective, efficient handling of these conditions is crucial in maintaining a safe environment. Tucci and colleagues[1,2] explain that a substantial proportion of ED visits are caused by mental health issues. In 2007, one in every eight ED visits involved a diagnosis related to a mental health or substance abuse condition. Strout and Baumann[3] found in a study of ED patients presenting with psychiatric complaints, that a diagnosis of schizophrenia or related psychotic disorder was a predictor of agitation. This article reviews the definitions of the term "psychosis." Possible causes of psychosis, including differential diagnoses, also are

This article is an update of an article previously published in Nursing Clinics of North America, Volume 38, Issue 1, March 2003.
[a] Office of Nursing Services, Veteran's Health Administration, 810 Vermont Avenue, Washington, DC 20420, USA; [b] Outpatient Mental Health, Salt Lake City VA Health Care System, 500 Foothill Boulevard, Salt Lake City, UT 84148, USA
* Corresponding author.
*E-mail address:* Lisa.Jensen@va.gov

considered. Treatment options and nursing interventions available in the ED are outlined.

## DEFINITIONS

The term "psychosis" brings to mind various images for clinicians. In general, an individual in a psychotic state is thought to be experiencing an impaired sense of reality. The Diagnostic and Statistical Manual of Mental Disorders–5th edition (DSM V)[4] states that psychotic disorders are defined as abnormalities in one of five domains. **Box 1** identifies those domains.

Wilson and Zeller[5] discuss the challenges of treating patients who present to the ED while undergoing a mental health crisis. These include dealing with several, often conflicting interests, such as police and legal issues, family wishes, patient advocates, and community wishes. Additionally, these patients present with psychiatric symptoms that may be caused by various medical conditions, substance intoxication or withdrawal, or psychiatric illnesses. Conceptually a patient with psychosis is thought to have a loss of ego boundaries or a gross impairment in reality testing. Allen[6] defined agitation as "a temporary disruption of typical physician-patient collaboration." He said that treatment decisions regarding an agitated patient must be made without any input from the patient, which is an "undesirable situation for all concerned."

An individual in a psychotic state can exhibit a variety of symptoms. Perceptual disturbances or hallucinatory experiences are often present in patients with schizophrenia or other psychotic disorders. The most common hallucinations are auditory, although patients also may experience visual, tactile, olfactory, and gustatory hallucinations. The auditory hallucinations or voices heard by a patient might be perceived by the patient as threatening, accusatory, or self-deprecating in nature. Birchwood and colleagues[7] describe a type of hallucination known as command hallucinations. They report that these hallucinations can be dangerous because individuals acting on them may put the public at risk for random acts of violence.

Delusional thinking is another hallmark of psychosis. According to Issacs[8] delusions are common symptoms of psychotic disorders and take a variety of forms. Emerging data also indicate that attributable bias (ie, self-serving) is a consistent characteristic of delusions.[9] Specifically, patients with delusions are likely to ascribe positive happenings to the self and negative happenings to external sources.[9]

One of the most common delusions is that of paranoia, characterized by suspiciousness and perceived persecution. Delusions also may be somatic in nature, with the belief that there is a problem with the functioning of one's body. Patients experiencing somatic delusions likely could present in the ED. Delusions also may be related to control of one's thinking. Patients may believe that thoughts are inserted into their minds, that their thoughts are broadcast to others, or that other people are able to control

---

**Box 1**
**Symptom domains of psychotic disorders**

Delusions

Hallucinations

Disorganized thinking (speech)

Negative symptoms

Grossly disorganized or abnormal motor behavior (including catatonia)

their thoughts. Disorganized speech and behavior also frequently are apparent in patients experiencing psychosis. When these are present, the patient may laugh inappropriately while conversing, or he or she may dress in inappropriate fashion.

## BEHAVIOR DISTURBANCES

Behavioral disturbances are common in patients with a psychotic disorder. The most serious behavioral disturbance exhibited by a patient with acute psychosis and agitation is that of aggression. An aggressive patient has the potential to cause physical harm to other patients in the ED and staff and visitors. In a study of nurses working in emergency settings, Cho and colleagues[10] found that 60% of participants experienced incidents of suspected abuse or violence. In addition, the aggressive patient could harm himself or herself or damage the facility.

Nurses working in the ED should be knowledgeable of what behavior may indicate potential physical disturbances. These behaviors include pacing in the waiting area; speaking with a raised voice or shouting; demanding to be seen immediately; threats of violence, which may be verbal or nonverbal; and escalation of any of these behaviors.

### Case Example

Family members bring a 42-year-old white man to the ED. The family reports that the man has been acting "strange" at home. He yells at the television when the news comes on, mutters to himself frequently, and insists on closing all of the blinds in the house during the day and night. The patient has a long history of psychiatric problems. He has been diagnosed in the past alternately as schizophrenia and bipolar. Now the patient is pacing about in the waiting area, looking down at the floor. His hands are at his sides, and he is clenching and unclenching his fists. He begins pacing at a quicker rate. He has been mumbling to himself. He now begins shouting a few words from time to time in addition to his muttering.

In the clinical example, immediate triaging and intervention with the patient are important for the safe management of this patient.

## ASSESSMENT AND DIAGNOSIS

Many psychiatric diagnoses can present as a threat to violence in the ED. An accurate diagnosis is essential in dealing appropriately with these patients. A patient who presents with agitation who is in a state of acute intoxication or withdrawal is treated differently than a patient experiencing an acute exacerbation of chronic schizophrenia or bipolar disorder–manic episode. It is important to determine the cause of the psychosis before determining the most practical and effective treatment. **Box 2** lists psychiatric diagnoses that may be seen in the ED.

---

**Box 2**
**Psychiatric diagnoses associated with agitation**

Brief psychotic episode

Bipolar disorder, manic phase

Schizoaffective disorder

Psychotic disorder caused by another medical condition

Acute intoxication

## Brief Psychotic Episode

The DSM V[4] defines "brief psychotic disorder" as including one or more of the following symptoms: hallucinations, delusions, disorganized speech, and grossly disorganized or catatonic behavior. It goes on to explain that brief psychotic disorder lasts more than 1 day and remits by 1 month. Saddock and colleagues[11] reported that individuals with brief psychotic disorder may have rapid shifts from one intense affect to another. They go on to state that although the disturbance may be short lived, the symptoms can be severe and the individual should be monitored closely to avoid potential harm to self and/or others.

## Schizophrenia

A patient with an acute exacerbation or first psychotic episode of schizophrenia often presents with similar positive symptoms as those exhibited by a patient experiencing a brief reactive psychosis. Although most patients with schizophrenia are not violent, Nielssen and colleagues[12] noted in a review of violence in patients experiencing a first episode of psychosis that one-third of them commit an act of violence before entering treatment. Of particular concern for staff in the ED is a patient with schizophrenia who is experiencing command hallucinations. The patient may hear voices telling him or her to harm specific types of people (ie, men with beards or young attractive women). The patient may believe he or she should direct that aggression toward people in general. The patient with schizophrenia with psychotic symptoms also could be experiencing visual hallucinations that may lead to violence. The patient might see another person as "the devil," which the patient perceives as a threat to be defended against or destroyed.

## Bipolar Disorder, Manic Phase

During a manic episode of bipolar disorder, the mood displayed can be expansive, irritable, grandiose, or elevated. The patient may present with an unusual appearance, in terms of clothing, grooming, and makeup. Speech may be loud and rapid, to the point that the listener is unable to understand the patient. Patients experiencing a manic phase describe the sensation of racing thoughts, which are not under their control. The heightened irritability often observed in the manic patient can result in violent behavior, particularly if the patient believes that he or she is being thwarted in attempts to obtain something or complete his or her perceived task.

## Schizoaffective Disorder

Patients showing symptoms that indicate a mood disorder in addition to psychotic symptoms are defined as having schizoaffective disorder. The mood symptoms seen in this disorder could be that of a depressed mood or manic symptoms. The DSM V[4] delineates that during an active phase of this illness, the diagnostic criteria for schizophrenia are met and the criteria for a major depressive episode or a manic episode.

## Psychotic Disorder Caused by Another Medical Condition

A patient presenting with a diagnosed medical condition who also is experiencing psychotic symptoms could meet the diagnostic criteria for psychotic disorder caused by another medical condition. The psychotic symptoms seen here are prominent hallucinations or delusions. Further criteria, according to the DSM V,[4] are evidence that the psychotic symptoms are judged to be attributable to the physiologic effects of another medical condition and not better explained by another mental disorder. Medical conditions that may result in a psychosis include, but are not limited to, cerebral tumors, epilepsy, migraine headaches, infections, endocrine and metabolic disorders, and hepatic or renal diseases.

### Acute Intoxication

Individuals present to the ED in various states of intoxication, with a variety of intoxicants. Phillips[13] found, through a literature review, that patients with schizophrenia often use substances to self-medicate their symptoms. A patient in a psychotic state also may present while acutely intoxicated with alcohol, to control his or her symptoms. Phillips also stated that psychostimulant drugs often are used to reduce negative symptoms, such as social withdrawal, whereas benzodiazepines and alcohol may be used to suppress temporarily positive symptoms, such as hallucinations.

Emerging data support implications from Phillips' study concerning the high use of substance use disorders in patients with schizophrenia. Researchers attribute assumptions about self-medication to findings from neuroimaging studies that implicate low striatal dopamine levels in patients with schizophrenia and related adverse side effects from antipsychotic medications. Increased substance use in patients with schizophrenia also increases psychosis.[14]

A person who is acutely intoxicated with alcohol may be belligerent and irritable on presentation. Patients undergoing detoxification may present to the ED with psychotic symptoms. Hallucinations, particularly visual and tactile, are common in individuals experiencing delirium tremens. Alcohol withdrawal symptoms, or delirium tremens, may occur within 1 week after the patient has stopped drinking, and the patient may not be acutely intoxicated. Assessment of alcohol intake and alcohol blood level is important because the treatment of an intoxicated patient is different from that of a patient who is acutely psychotic without having ingested any alcohol or mood-altering drugs.

Patients taking illicit drugs also can present in an agitated, psychotic state. These patients may not have a history of a psychotic disorder. Use of cocaine can result in a state of intense paranoia. The use of hallucinogens often results in the experience of intense hallucinations. Friends or family members, who could be unaware of any drugs that have been ingested, may bring patients to the ED. Patients may be unwilling to admit to the use of the drugs because of their illicit nature. With any patient in whom there is a suspicion of drug use, a toxicology screen is indicated.

### Differential Diagnosis

Determining the correct diagnosis when treating an agitated patient with psychosis is essential in deciding on the most appropriate treatment. Delirium often is the cause of perceptual disturbances experienced by patients. Delirium usually is noted by a sudden onset of symptoms. The DSM V[4] describes delirium as being a disturbance in attention that develops over a short period of time, usually hours to a few days. Patients experiencing a delirium generally present with confusion and disorientation, hallucinations, and often unusual behaviors. The delirious state may be interposed throughout the day with periods of lucidity.

There are many possible physiologic causes of delirium, including systemic infections, cardiovascular conditions, metabolic disorder, drug toxicity, or a nutritional disorder. Patients with other medical disorders also may present to the ED in an agitated state. A patient with a closed head injury could be agitated, anxious, and possibly experiencing hallucinations. Determining the cause is important in selecting the most appropriate treatment and management. A comprehensive history and physical examination that includes diagnostic studies, such as fluid and electrolytes, hematologic, renal and hepatic studies, drug screens, urinalysis, and endocrines studies is an essential component of making a differential diagnosis and initiating appropriate interventions.

Equally important is conducting a psychosocial assessment that includes questions about current prescribed, over-the-counter and herbal preparations with psychoactive properties. Because acute psychosis interferes with the patient's concentration and thought processes it is important to collect data from family members, other providers, and significant others. The assessment also needs to include a mental status examination, presence and history of suicidal thoughts and attempts and violence, and substance use history.

## TREATMENT AND INTERVENTIONS

It is estimated that mental health presentations account for about 6% to 9% of all ED visits.[15] Many of these patients exhibit agitated behavior secondary to psychosis. Most EDs do not have separate psychiatric emergency services, thus treatment and interventions for acute psychosis present significant challenges for the ED staff. The nurse plays a central role in all phases of treatment of the agitated patient with acute psychosis. The nurse is responsible for ensuring the safe management of the patient, and also ensuring the security and safety of the ED environment for other patients, their family members, and staff. Assessment begins immediately when the nurse observes the behavior exhibited by the patient as the triage process is initiated. All emergent medical and psychiatric needs must be attended to immediately, including vital sign abnormalities, wounds, and agitated behavior.

The patient who is acutely agitated and psychotic can escalate rapidly while in the waiting area before triage. **Box 3** outlines behaviors commonly seen in patients with agitation and acute psychosis. Observation for the presence of hallucinations might reveal facial expressions indicating the patient is listening to, or responding internally to voices. The patient might verbally respond and converse with the voices, or may look for the origin of the voices by glancing over their shoulder or by turning around to see if someone is behind them. Documentation in the medical record should contain descriptions of the behaviors observed, and include the general appearance of the patient, grooming, and the manner of dress.

As the nurse moves to the interview phase of the assessment, it is important to provide a private area to ensure confidentiality for the patient as long as the safety of the patient, the staff, and other patients in the ED is not jeopardized. This may require having another staff member or security stand by in close proximity during

---

**Box 3**
**Common behaviors of agitated patients with psychosis**

Pacing

Invading other's space

Hypersexual behavior

Abnormal gait

Speaking loudly or inappropriately

Removing clothing

Marching in place

Exhibit unusual stationary postures

the interview process. Informing the patient of such necessary safety requirements in a matter of fact approach likely enhances cooperation with the interview process. Using a direct interview style while eliciting information regarding the presence of auditory hallucinations is preferred. Inquiring about the number of different voices the patient is hearing, whether the voices are recognized by the patient, the frequency, intensity, duration, and content of the hallucinations are all important pieces of information in the evaluation process. If there are additional hallucinations or perceptual disturbances being experienced, they are evaluated in the same way. The patient's perceived emotional response to hallucinations should also be noted. According to Moller,[16] careful observation and practiced active listening skills enhance the assessment accuracy and likelihood of successful interventions with the patient experiencing hallucinations.

### Safety

Provision of a safe environment is a primary consideration when a patient who is acutely agitated and psychotic is receiving treatment in the ED. Nurses play a principal role in ensuring the environment is safe. Being respectful of the patient's personal space helps ensure the safety of staff approaching the patient. A patient who is agitated often believes he or she is being threatened and may strike out to protect himself or herself. The patient is more likely to respond cooperatively when approached with a calm manner and voice. The nurse should guard against facing the patient directly when talking with him or her; it is better to stand at an angle, which prevents the patient from feeling trapped, and allows for a quick escape from the situation should the need arise. If a staff member is alone in a room with a patient who is agitated, the staff member needs to ensure personal safety by sitting near the closest exit. Objects that can be picked up easily and thrown about the room should be removed or kept at a minimum (see **Box 5**).

### Therapeutic Alliance

The formation of a therapeutic alliance is necessary to manage the psychiatric patient effectively.[17] Frequently, the relationship formed with the patient is the primary intervention tool that is used for successful outcomes. A high level of trust is necessary for the patient to feel safe to open up to the nurse and reveal symptoms being experienced. Patients with acute psychosis as a rule understand that what they are experiencing is unusual. They may be reluctant to share information for fear of being humiliated. A patient who is paranoid and suspicious may believe that he or she can trust no one or may think that he or she has information that can be shared only with particular individuals. Approaching the patient with a nonjudgmental attitude is crucial to the formation of a therapeutic alliance. Arguing with a patient about their paranoid thoughts, delusional thinking, or hallucinations may increase anxiety and agitation and interferes with establishing a trusting relationship. The best approach is to acknowledge the patient's experience and ask the patient how he or she is feeling emotionally about the symptoms from which he or she is suffering.

### Case Example

A 30-year-old male patient presents to the ED requesting renewal of his psychotropic medication and insisting it is the responsibility of the hospital to provide free medication for him to his take to his residential care facility. He informs the nurse that he "owns the hospital" and will have her fired if she does not get a doctor immediately to prescribe and dispense his medication to him. He states he has not had his medication for close to a month and is going to be evicted from the care facility very soon if he does not get back on his medication. He becomes increasingly agitated, pacing back and forth in the interview room, his voice getting louder as he continues to threaten the nurse with her job. A therapeutic response would be for the nurse to say, "I can see why you are upset and frustrated, it must be difficult for you to go without your medication when you are aware how important they are to your health. Would you be willing to have a seat, and I can have the doctor come in to review your medications so you can start taking them again?"

It is important to convey that you want to help and to realize that the patient feels out of control. This experience is frightening to the patient and his verbally aggressive behavior is an attempt to gain some control. Exhibiting a calm demeanor and validating his frustration enables the patient to move toward regaining control and to relax in a calm, safe environment.

### Provision of a Calm Environment

Providing the patient with acute agitation and psychosis with a quiet, calm environment is essential in the practical management of the patient. Placing the patient in a private examination room, if available, is indicated. Having the same staff members interact with the patient decreases confusion for him or her. The use of direct, simple messages and nonconfrontational feedback is encouraged when interacting with individuals suffering with psychotic symptoms.[18] The use of limited choices is suggested (ie, "would you prefer to sit in the chair or lay on the exam table?"). Offering choices gives the patient a sense of control in the situation. Minimizing the noise level also contributes to calming the patient. Available family members or other support persons may be able to assist in decreasing discomfort for the patient. Family members and caregivers may also be a source of agitation in some patients with acute psychosis, so it is important to observe the patient's response to family involvement.

### Use of Medications

Medications are often used to manage psychotic, agitated behavior in the ED. Commonly used medications are listed in **Box 4**. These include benzodiazepines (eg, lorazepam) and antipsychotics (eg, haloperidol). In recent years, several studies have also shown increased safety and agitation control from atypical antipsychotics, especially in persons with a known psychotic disorder.

Multiple studies have shown the efficacy of benzodiazepines for acute agitation and sedation. In addition, some evidence indicates that patients with unknown causes of agitation or causes secondary to alcohol intoxication or withdrawal have better results and fewer adverse effects using benzodiazepines alone compared with benzodiazepines in combination with antipsychotics or antipsychotics alone.

Lorazepam seems to be a good rational choice when treating an acute episode of agitation, especially when the cause is not clear. Lorazepam is a nonspecific sedating

---

**Box 4**
**Medications commonly used for agitation**

- Benzodiazepines (lorazepam)

- Antipsychotics (haloperidol)

- Atypical antipsychotics
  - Risperidone
  - Aripiprazole
  - Ziprasidone
  - Olanzapine

benzodiazepine. Lorazepam has been shown to be at least as effective as haloperidol in controlling violent behavior.[19] Of the available benzodiazepines, lorazepam is the only one reliably absorbed when administered intramuscularly. Because of this property, it is most often the benzodiazepine of choice for agitated patients in the ED. Its half-life is relatively short (10–20 h), and it has no active metabolites. The usual dosage of 0.5 to 2 mg every 1 to 6 hours may be administered orally, sublingually, intramuscularly, or intravenously. Caution is required when respiratory depression is a possibility, despite lorazepam being less of a problem than with agents previously popular before its advent. Nevertheless, patients at risk for respiratory depression should be monitored carefully. Other adverse effects include hypotension and extreme somnolence. Clonazepam is another benzodiazepine that might be used to treat agitation; it is absorbed quickly, but does have a longer half-life than lorazepam. It is used in oral form, tablet or sublingual.

Conventional or typical antipsychotics include the butyrophenones and phenothiazines. By far the most common of the typical antipsychotics used for acute agitation, violent behavior, and psychosis is haloperidol. Haloperidol has been used for years, either by mouth or intramuscularly, to control violence and acute psychosis. Disruptive behavior has been shown to be alleviated using haloperidol within 30 minutes for most patients who present to the ED with acute agitation from various causes. The onset of haloperidol intramuscularly or intravenously is approximately 30 to 45 minutes, although it may take up to 60 minutes in some patients. Although other more sedating typical antipsychotics, such as chlorpromazine, were previously used, side effects, such as orthostatic hypotension, limited widespread use with favor going to haloperidol.

Droperidol is another typical antipsychotic in the butyrophenone class; its use is most often limited to induction of anesthesia. The medication is not approved by the Food and Drug Administration for psychiatric conditions but has been used for sedating agitated patients in ED settings. It has a black box warning in the United States because of the possibility of prolongation of the QT interval and subsequent risk of fatal arrhythmia (torsades de pointes). It is no longer available in the United Kingdom. Use of haloperidol or droperidol requires monitoring for possible side effects. Extrapyramidal symptoms (EPS) are common with these medications. The EPS concern in this setting includes dystonia, akathisia, and parkinsonism symptoms. Dystonia encompasses a wide array of symptoms; the most frightening for the patient are oral spasms, laryngospasm, and oculogyric crisis. The patient actually loses voluntary control of muscles when any of these side effects occur. Parkinsonism symptoms include stiffness, masklike facies, and shuffling gait. The most common complaint with akathisia includes inner restlessness, jitteriness, difficulty sitting still, and fidgeting. Acute-onset EPS are most common during early treatment with these mediations.[20]

The nurse's role in monitoring for potential side effects when these medications are administered is an additional challenge. When these side effects emerge, as they often do, treatment requires administration of diphenhydramine or benztropine mesylate for rapid and effective treatment either intramuscularly or intravenously.

There have been a few randomized trials indicating the combination of a benzodiazepine with a traditional or classic antipsychotic results in a more rapid onset of sedation with a similar adverse effect profile. Extrapyramidal adverse effects are exhibited at a slightly higher rate when an antipsychotic only is used than when a combination is administered. Combination therapy, such as lorazepam and haloperidol, is considered standard practice to control agitation in an acute setting.

Atypical antipsychotic agents approved for intramuscular injection include ziprasidone for use in agitation associated with schizophrenia, and olanzapine intramuscular and aripiprazole intramuscular for use in agitation associated with either schizophrenia or bipolar mania.[20,21] The atypical antipsychotics have a much more favorable side effect profile than the typical antipsychotics. EPS side effects are rare with the atypical agents although still a possibility.

Intramuscular injection has a faster onset of action and predictable course than oral administration; however, a patient may calm down readily after an oral dose because he or she realizes that action has been taken and help is being provided. Sublingual administration may have a faster onset of action than oral ingestion and has the added advantage of distracting the agitated patient while the pill is dissolving. Risperidone was one of the first atypical antipsychotics on the market and has also been shown to be as efficacious in treating psychosis and agitation as haloperidol, with significantly fewer adverse effects. The use of atypical antipsychotics in combination with lorazepam is a choice that is also at times used by ED staff with good result in the patient with acute agitation and psychosis. Although the administration of medication is widely used to manage agitation and psychosis, equally important is the implementation of psychosocial interventions that convey empathy and support and ensure patient and staff safety.

### Verbal De-Escalation

Nurses working in the ED or other high-risk areas must be clinically skilled and competent in de-escalation techniques. Most organizations and accreditation organizations (ie, Joint Commission) require that all staff receive a minimum of annual training on verbal de-escalation, and a higher level of training is indicated when staff works on acute psychiatric inpatient units or high-risk areas. During these potentially violent situations it is imperative for nurses and other staff to use the least restrictive approach and use verbal de-escalation techniques.[22] **Box 5** provides specific techniques to ensure staff safety and verbal de-escalation techniques.

### Seclusion and Restraint

There are rare occasions when interventions to decrease agitation are not successful and a severely agitated patient may require physical restraint. Using seclusion and

---

**Box 5**
**Ensure staff safety: verbal de-escalation**

| Ensure Staff Safety | Limit Setting |
|---|---|
| • Maintain a safe distance | • Use when *more control* is needed |
| • Establish rapport; reassure and support | • Should be *appropriate* to circumstances |
| • Stand on nondominant side | • Be clear, *direct*, and supportive |
| • Use nonthreatening body language | • Show *respect* for others |
| • Avoid glaring eye contact, pointing, or touching | • Give *options* if possible |
| • Give information in terms of a suggestion, rather than instruction | • State *consequences* if necessary |
| • Remove anything from your person that can be used as a weapon or can be grabbed | • Seek to maintain *personal dignity* and therapeutic relationships |
| • Pay attention to your "gut feeling" | |
| • Redirect | |

*From* Antai-Otong D. Psychiatric emergencies. Eau Claire (WI): PESI; 2009; with permission.

| **Box 6** |
|---|
| **Documentation requirements for restraint usage** |
| Reasons for restraining a patient (patient/staff safety and protection) |
| Type of restraint used (eg, locked room vs four-point leather) |
| Maximum duration of restraint |
| Alternate less restrictive interventions attempted |

restraints to manage an out of control patient situation must be the last alternative, specifically after attempts to verbally de-escalate the situation fail.

Proper physical restraints and individuals trained in their application should be available at all times in the ED. **Box 6** outlines documentation requirements for restrain usage. Most EDs are limited to restraints because seclusion rooms are rarely available in EDs. Restraints limit physical mobility, whereas seclusion involves containment, isolation, and a decrease in sensory input. The patient must be monitored continuously while restrained physically. Restraint and seclusion orders are to be renewed at regular intervals not to exceed 4 hours.

It is critical when using seclusion and restraint interventions for staff to be familiar with ED and hospital regulations, and Joint Commission and other accrediting agency guidelines, regional statues, and federal law. Requirements regarding the use of physical restraints, containment (seclusion), psychiatric commitment, and transfers of care are monitored closely by government agencies and accrediting bodies. Because of the risks inherent in use of this intervention, there should be frequent facility oversight of the process, policy, and training.[23]

In most cases, chemical restraint (ie, sedation) is preferable to physical restraint when prolonged behavioral control is necessary or when the patient is severely combative. Any physical restraint of a combative patient can lead to serious injury or death (eg, from aspiration, sudden cardiac death, rhabdomyolysis) and as such should be avoided whenever feasible.

### Debriefing Staff Members

The use of restraints is controversial and should be used as a last resort in the management of violent behavior. Placing an individual in restraints can be a traumatic experience for all involved. A short debriefing session can be a meaningful component of the intervention. Debriefing gives the staff time to express their feelings and reaction to the situation. It also allows the team an opportunity to discuss what went right and what could have been improved on during the intervention.

Intervening with a patient with acute agitation and psychosis in the ED is a challenge for even the most skilled clinician. Making an accurate assessment initially assists the staff in selecting the most appropriate disposition for the patient. Providing care to these patients in a safe manner is also an important element in their treatment. Nurses in the ED play a key role in ensuring the safe, efficient, compassionate treatment of the psychotic, agitated patient.

### SUMMARY

Patients experiencing acute psychosis often present to EDs. Management of acute agitation and psychosis can be a challenge for the staff. Medical stabilization, appropriate assessment, and diagnosis are important. Verbal de-escalation and other psychosocial interventions are helpful in creating a safe and therapeutic environment.

Psychiatric and emergency room nurses are poised to treat patients presenting with acute psychosis and must be knowledgeable of evidence-based approaches to treat these complex disorders.

## REFERENCES

1. Kuo DC, Tucci V. The hidden costs of behavioral and psychiatric emergencies. Emerg Med Clin North Am 2015;33:xvii–xviii.
2. Owens PL, Mutter R, Stocks C. Mental health and substance abuse-related emergency department visits among adults, 2007: Statistical Brief #92. AHRQ H.CUP. 2010.
3. Strout TD, Baumann MR. Agitation in the emergency department: importance of schizophrenia and related disorders. Ann Emerg Med 2015;66(4 Suppl):S145.
4. American Psychiatric Association. Diagnostic and statistical manual of mental disorders. 5th edition. Arlington (VA): American Psychiatric Publishing; 2013.
5. Wilson MP, Zeller SL. Introduction: reconsidering psychiatry in the emergency room. J Emerg Med 2012;5:771–2.
6. Allen MH. Managing the agitated psychotic patient: a reappraisal of the evidence. J Clin Psychiatry 2000;61(Suppl 14):11–20.
7. Birchwood M, Michail M, Meadon A, et al. Cognitive behavior therapy to prevent harmful compliance with command hallucinations (COMMAND): a randomized controlled trial. Lancet Psychiatry 2014;1:23–33.
8. Issacs A. Mental health and psychiatric nursing. 4th edition. Philadelphia: Lippincott Williams & Wilkins; 2005. p. 122.
9. So SH, Tang V, Leung PW. Dimensions of delusions and attribution biases along the continuum of psychosis. PLoS One 2015;10:e0144558.
10. Cho OH, Cha KS, Yoo YS. Awareness and attitudes towards violence and abuse among emergency nurses. Asian Nurs Res (Korean Soc Nurs Sci) 2015;9:213–8.
11. Sadock BJ, Sadock VA, Ruiz P. Kaplan & Sadock's synopsis of psychiatry: behavior sciences/clinical psychiatry. 11th edition. Philadelphia: Lippincott Williams & Wilkins; 2014. p. 339–42.
12. Nielssen OB, Malhi GS, McGorry PD. Overview of violence to self and others during the first episode of psychosis. J Clin Psychiatry 2012;73:e580–7.
13. Phillips P. Substance misuse, offending and mental illness: a review. J Psychiatr Ment Health Nurs 2000;7:483–9.
14. Award AG, Voruganti LL. Revisiting the 'self-medication' hypothesis in light of the new data linking low striatal dopamine to comorbid addictive behavior. Ther Adv Psychopharmacol 2015;5:172–8.
15. Hazlett SB, McCarthy ML, Londner MS, et al. Epidemiology of adult psychiatric visits to US emergency departments. Acad Emerg Med 2008;11(2):193–5.
16. Moller MD. Neurobiological responses to schizophrenia and other psychotic disorders. In: Stuart G, Laraia M, editors. Principles and practices of psychiatric nursing. 8th edition. St Louis (MO): CV Mosby; 2005. p. 355.
17. Nordstrom K, Zun LS, Wilson MP, et al. Medical evaluation and triage of the agitated patient: consensus statement of the American Association for Emergency Psychiatry project Beta medical evaluation workgroup. West J Emerg Med 2012;13:3–10.
18. Vass V, Morrison AP, Law H, et al. How stigma impacts on people with psychosis: the mediating effect of self-esteem and hopelessness on subjective recovery and psychotic experiences. Psychiatry Res 2015;230:26–34.

19. Wilson MP, Minassian A, Bahramzi M, et al. Despite expert recommendations, second-generation antipsychotics are not often prescribed in the emergency department. J Emerg Med 2014;46:808–13.
20. American Psychiatric Association. Practice guideline for the treatment of patients with schizophrenia. 2nd edition. Arlington (VA): American Psychiatric Association Publishing; 2010.
21. Wilson MP, Pepper D, Currier GW, et al. The psychopharmacology of agitation: consensus statement of the American Association for Emergency Psychiatry project Beta psychopharmacology workgroup. West J Emerg Med 2012;13:26–34.
22. Antai-Otong D. Psychiatric emergencies. Eau Claire (WI): PESI; 2009.
23. Joint Commission Resources. Approved: standards revisions addressing patient flow through the emergency department. Jt Comm Perspect 2012;32:1–5.

# Treatment Approaches to Attention Deficit Hyperactivity Disorder

Deborah Antai-Otong, MS, APRN, PMHCNS-BC, FAAN[a],
Michele L. Zimmerman, MA, PMHCNS-BC[b,c],*

## KEYWORDS

- Neurodevelopmental disorders • Psychostimulants • Psychoeducation
- Attention deficit hyperactivity disorder

## KEY POINTS

- Attention deficit hyperactivity disorder (ADHD) is a very common disorder that originates in childhood but persists into adulthood.
- Multimodal treatment demonstrates the most promising clinical outcomes for patients with ADHD.
- ADHD impacts entire families and communities.

## INTRODUCTION

Attention- Deficit/ Hyperactivity disorder (ADHD) formerly was classified as a Disruptive Behavior Disorder. However, it is now recognized as a Neurodevelopmental Disorder, which takes it out of the realm of behavior disorder. As a neurodevelopmental disorder, it has onset in the developmental period, which manifest often prior to the child beginning grade school. These disorders produce impairments in personal, social, academic or occupational functional.[1] ADHD is a common neurodevelopmental disorder in children, adolescents, and adults, with the prevalence estimated to range from 5% to 7% across cultures[2,3] and approximately 2% to 5% in adults.[2,4] The prevalence is 5.4 million children and 10.3 million adults and is estimated to occur in most

Disclosures: None.
This article is an update of an article previously published in *Nursing Clinics of North America*, Volume 38, Issue 1, March 2003.
[a] Department of Veterans Affairs, Veterans Integrated Service Networks-(VISN-17), 2301 E. Lamar Boulevard, Arlington, TX 76006, USA; [b] Finney Zimmerman Psychiatric Associates PLC, 324 Louisa Avenue Suite 125, Virginia Beach, VA 23454, USA; [c] Psychiatric Nursing, Old Dominion University, 5115 Hampton Boulevard, Norfolk, VA 23529, USA
* Corresponding author. Finney Zimmerman Psychiatric Associates PLC, 324 Louisa Avenue Suite 125, Virginia Beach, VA 23454.
*E-mail address:* mzimmerman@psych-therapy.com

cultures.[5] Data from a recent study involving self-reports from parents indicate that ADHD has increased by 43% across all cultures and ethnicities since 2011 and that 1 in 8 children and adolescents had a diagnosis of this disorder.[6] Among children, the gender ratio is 3:1 boys to girls, and among adults, the gender ratio is 2:1 or lower. It seems that more girls and women than boys and men have the inattentive subtype. Symptoms of ADHD are likely to originate by age 12[2,7] and continue through adulthood.

ADHD is highly influenced by genetic liability.[8,9] Researchers assert that the genetic vulnerability to ADHD is linked to rare aberrations and vast genes that influence neuro-transmission and neurodevelopmental pathways.[10] Children and adolescents with ADHD are highly likely to have a coexisting psychiatric or substance use disorder, such as oppositional defiant disorder, conduct disorder, mood disorders, anxiety disorders, Tourette disorder, chronic tic disorders, learning and language disorders, and substance abuse in adolescents.[7,11,12] Essential features of ADHD include a persistent pattern of inattention, hyperactivity/impulsivity, or combined symptoms and severity and impairment than those typically observed in individuals at a comparable level of development.[7] Classification of these clusters may be mild, moderate, or severe depending on the level of symptom severity.[7]

Nurses in vast clinical and community practice settings should be able to recognize symptoms of ADHD and clinical challenges associated with these lifelong and complex disorders. Psychiatric nurses must be familiar with the course of ADHD in children, adolescents, and adults and knowledgeable of person-centered and evidence-based treatment that helps these patients and their families optimize academic and functional performance. This article overviews core features of ADHD and underlying causative factors that are targets for multimodal treatment. It further emphasizes the importance of data collection primarily from the patient,and significant others, in adults. For children and adolescents, parents and teachers are the primary providers of information necessary for diagnosis. The role of the nurse in the identification, assessment, and treatment of patients and their families with ADHD is also discussed.

## CORE FEATURES

The Diagnostic and Statistical Manual of Mental Disorders, 5th edition (DSM-5)[7] delineates the 3 core features of ADHD as inattention, hyperactivity-impulsivity, and combined type. Symptoms must persist for at least 6 months, be observed before age 12, and produce considerable global functional disturbances. This disorder is also likely to result in the following behaviors:

- Impaired response inhibition, impulse control, or the capacity to delay gratification
- Excessive task-irrelevant activity of activity poorly regulated to the demands of a situation ("on the go")
- Poor sustained attention or persistence of effort to tasks. Individuals have difficulty with tedious or protracted tasks, completing routine assignments, and working independently
- Difficulty remembering to do things or poor working memory
- Delayed development of internal language (the mind's voice) and rule-following
- Difficulties with regulation of emotions, motivation, and arousal
- Diminished problem-solving ability, ingenuity, and flexibility in pursuing long-term goals
- Greater than normal variability in task or work performance[13,14]

## CAUSATIVE FACTORS

Although the precise cause of ADHD continues to be researched, there are convincing data that implicate vast brain structures, neurochemistry, and genetic and environmental factors as key contributors to these neurodevelopmental disorders.

### Neurochemical and Neuroanatomical

The underlying cause of ADHD is obscure, although there is growing evidence that links it with biologic, genetic, neuroanatomic, and environmental factors. Enormous progress continues to be made concerning the cause of ADHD. Neurobiologic theories include dysregulation of complex biochemical processes and genetic variants involving dopaminergic and noradrenergic systems and neural pathways.[15–17] Specifically, pharmacologic studies indicate the efficacy of psychostimulants and modulation of certain dopamine systems. Additional studies implicate alterations in dopamine systems in the role of persistence, distractibility, motivation, and motor control.[18] Inadequate modulation or hyperactivation of norepinephrine systems is thought to contribute to hyperactivity and inattentiveness, core features of ADHD.

Neuroimaging studies indicate reduced profusion in frontal and temporal lobes and the dopamine-concentrated basal ganglia regions to self-regulation disturbances in children with ADHD. These studies further implicate these brain regions in the development of cognitive disturbances that affect concentration, arousal, and motivation.[19,20] Long term studies beginning during pregnancy indicate that mothers with perinatal mood and anxiety disorders have are more likely to have children with ADHD, Oppositional Defiant Disorder as well as depression and anxiety by age 8 (Women's Health, the Journal of the Marce Society).

### Genetics

Voluminous research strongly supports the role of genetic and familial patterns in the development of ADHD. Twin studies indicate high heritability of ADHD that ranges from 70% to 80%, whereas data from adult samples indicate moderate incidence of 30% to 40%.[16,17,21] There is growing interest in the heritability of ADHD in adults, but less data are available concerning the genetic basis of ADHD in adults mainly due to a lack of methodological issues (ie, age-specific assessment tools).[10,15] Data also demonstrate structural alterations that are consistent in children and their parents, further strengthening support of the role of genetics and familial influences.[16,22–24]

### Environmental

The most common environmental factors associated with ADHD stem from pregnancy and delivery-related complications, including traumatic brain injury and low birth weight. Other possible causes include various agents that can lead to brain injury or abnormal brain development, such as fetal exposure to alcohol and tobacco, severe early childhood deprivation, childhood exposures to streptococcal infection, early exposure to high levels of lead and household gas.[22,25–27] Prenatal and postnatal primary prevention and education about the dangers of modifiable risk factors, such as alcohol and tobacco, offer opportunities for nurses to mitigate environmental factors linked to ADHD.

Nurses working with patients with ADHD and their caregivers must be able to integrate basic biologic factors into the assessment process and treatment planning. Of particular importance is the recognition of behaviors that reflect altered neurobiologic processes, determine appropriate interventions, and educate the patient and caregivers about this common, chronic, and disabling psychiatric disorder. Diagnosis of ADHD requires comprehensive data collection from various sources, including the patient, caregivers or family members, teachers, and employers.

## DIAGNOSIS, ASSESSMENT, AND EVALUATION

The comprehensive biopsychosocial assessment process begins with the establishment of rapport with the child, adolescent, or adult, family member, and significant others. Because of the high incidence of coexisting psychiatric disorders, such as depression, the nurse must also conduct a risk assessment for suicide and other self-destructive behaviors. (See Ramirez J: Suicide: Across the Life Span, in this issue.)

As previously noted, the assessment process must be comprehensive and include data from many sources. During this process, the nurse is also challenged to identify and assess core features of ADHD—inattention, hyperactivity, and impulsivity—to meet DSM-5 criteria.[7]

Normally, the biopsychosocial assessment involves input from various sources and often begins with the parent interview. During this interview, the parent self-reports the onset, duration, and impact of symptoms on the family. Initially, the nurse may gather data from parents or caregivers regarding the core symptoms of ADHD in various settings, the age of onset, duration of symptoms, and degree of functional impairment or problem behaviors and nature of family relationships. Equally important is the identification of the family's chief concerns, including a history of signs and symptoms. Asking questions about the family's history of learning difficulties, smoking, and substance use especially during pregnancy, along with questions about mood disorders, and their own school, and occupational experiences, help the nurse identify risk factors associated with the child's disorder.[12] Verbal narratives, written narratives, questionnaires, and rating scales are essential, and the use of global clinical impressions or general descriptions within domains of attention and activity is insufficient to diagnose ADHD.

Interviewing the child alone is not sufficient because children lack insight into their behaviors. It is essential to glean data and necessary to use direct information from multiple informants, such as teacher report forms, report cards, attendance records, and information from coaches and other significant adults. According to the American Academy of Pediatrics,[12] because of the high prevalence of co-occurrence of other psychiatric disorders and possible physical causes of ADHD, it is imperative that the patient is medically cleared and a differential diagnosis is determined before initiation of treatment. **Table 1** lists conditions that may mimic symptoms of this ADHD. It is also necessary to obtain evidence directly from the classroom teacher about core symptoms, duration, impairment, and coexisting conditions. The American Academy of Pediatrics recommends that physicians review these reports, which should include verbal narratives, written narratives, questionnaires, or rating scales. Teachers are not licensed or educated, however, to make a diagnosis of ADHD, and they may not make a recommendation that a child receive treatment—medicine or other treatment—for ADHD.[12,28]

Other assessment tools include rating scales and information from academic and employment function. Standardized rating scales are an important component of the assessment and may be used by trained therapists or other certified instructors and other mental health professionals making a differential diagnosis of ADHD. Barkley[13,14] checklists and rating scales are used widely to make a correct diagnosis and guide behavioral and psychosocial planning. Other tools include the Achenbach

**Table 1**
**Differential diagnosis of attention deficit hyperactivity disorder**

| General Medical Conditions | Psychiatric Disorders | Environmental Factors |
|---|---|---|
| • Hyperthyroidism | • Bipolar disorders | • Stressful family environment |
| • Sleep disorders | • Depression | • Poor parenting skills |
| • Medication side effects (ie, bronchodilators, antipsychotics, thyroid replacement hormones, anticonvulsants) | • Dysthymic disorder | • Untreated parental psychiatric disorders |
| | • Posttraumatic stress disorder | • Child abuse/neglect |
| | • Oppositional defiant disorder | • Dysfunctional family systems |
| • Lead toxicity | • Intermittent explosive disorder | • Lack of academic understanding and supportive services children/ adolescent and families |
| • Seizure disorders | • Specific learning disorder | |
| • Neurodevelopmental disorders, such as intellectual disability disorder | • Autism spectrum disorder | |
| | • Substance use disorder | |
| | • Personality disorder, such as antisocial disorder | • Social disadvantage and poverty |
| • Fetal alcohol syndrome | | |
| • Hearing and/or visual impairments | | • School sector, location, size, and school socioeconomic |

Note: It is imperative to conduct the following studies before initiating stimulants: 1. serum complete blood count with differential; 2. electrolyte levels; 3. liver function tests (before initiation of stimulant therapy); 4. thyroid function tests.
*Data from* Refs.[7,12,13,28]

Child Behavior Checklist[29] and the Conner Abbreviated Teacher Rating Scale.[30] Structured behavioral observations in naturalistic and other settings are helpful in measuring medication response and yielding data regarding the teacher's management style.

## COURSE OF ATTENTION DEFICIT HYPERACTIVITY DISORDER

Historically, ADHD was thought to be a childhood disorder that affected children and adolescents and their families. More recent studies confirm that the course and developmental risk of ADHD persists through adulthood and contributes to lifelong impaired academic, occupational, and social functioning, independent of conduct-related problems and coexisting psychiatric, substance use and physical disorders.[31,32] More than 70% of hyperactive children continue to meet criteria for ADHD during adolescence, and 65% of teens may continue to meet the criteria for this disorder in adulthood. Kessler and his colleagues[33] concluded that executive function symptoms are more prominent in adults than children and adolescents with ADHD. These assertions suggest that adults with ADHD are more likely to exhibit inattentiveness and less hyperactivity and impulsivity when compared with younger age groups. Clinical implications from these findings suggest that ADHD symptoms vary over time.

Common adult behaviors associated with ADHD[7,11] include the following:

- Inability to relax—motor hyperactivity
- Attention deficits—easily distracted, difficulty maintaining concentrations on activities, such as reading
- Affective lability—dating back to adolescence (ie, boredom, depressed)
- Hot temper, explosive behaviors—"short fuse," "easily rattled"
- Overreactivity—inappropriate expression of anger, "stressed out"

- Disorganization—poor time-management skills
- Impulsive behaviors—using poor judgment, such as speaking before thinking about consequences
- Interpersonal, academic, and occupational disturbances

As a result of these behaviors, adults with ADHD are likely to be undereducated relative to their intellectual ability and family educational background. They experience difficulties with work adjustment and may be underemployed in their occupations relative to their intelligence and educational and family backgrounds. They experience problems resulting from procrastination, lack of productivity, and disorganization. They have a tendency to be scattered and lack effective time management skills. The impulsive blurting out that is characteristic of the disorder is often unsuitable to appropriate workplace behavior. They "tune out" during instructional situations, on-the-job training sessions, or meetings and have difficulty following instructions.

Additional behaviors in the patient with ADHD include making piles of materials and files and having difficulty finding things. They experience fidgetiness and edginess, difficulty following instructions and listening, problems interrupting and intruding on others, and creating distress in others. They are likely to be fired and tend to change their jobs more often because of boredom or interpersonal problems. They are more likely to report a history of unstable or chaotic relationships, marital discord, and divorce. Adults with ADHD also have troubles with traffic violations and resultant accidents and the prospect of license suspension. Frequently, this population is eligible for reasonable accommodations in their workplace or educational settings under the Americans with Disabilities Act, provided that the severity of the ADHD is such that it produces impairments in one or more major areas of life functioning and that they disclose their disorder to their employer or educational institution.[34]

## TREATMENT CONSIDERATIONS

Once a diagnosis of ADHD is confirmed, the nurse should seek consent from the parent or caregiver and discuss treatment considerations with the patient, family, and teacher. During this discussion, the nurse must also explain the diagnosis, symptoms, and related impairment, and academic needs and treatment options.[30] Treatment considerations need to be person-centered and based on the patient and family's wishes, strengths, preferences, and needs. Failure to treat ADHD is likely to have extensive and negative consequences.

It is well documented that the most effective treatment approach is multimodal, person-centered, strength-based, and comprehensive and integrates pharmacologic and psychotherapeutic interventions. ADHD practice guidelines suggest that multimodal approaches need to include behavioral treatment, medications, and parental training to optimize mental health, quality of life, and functioning.[28] Specific treatment targets include moderating inattentiveness, hyperactivity, impulsivity, and ameliorating psychosocial and academic and occupational performance and parenting skills.[35]

Multimodal treatment focus must also address the needs and concerns of family members and caregivers who may present with high levels of distress and incidence of psychiatric disorders, such as depression.[36] Failure to address the needs of family members of patients with ADHD is likely to result in poor treatment outcomes and persistent academic and occupational performance challenges across the lifespan.

## PHARMACOTHERAPY

An in-depth discussion of pharmacologic interventions used to treat ADHD is beyond the scope of this article. The next sections center on major drugs used to treatment these disorders.

The decision to medicate is based on a definitive diagnosis of ADHD and persistent core symptoms that are sufficiently severe to cause functional and social impairment at school and usually at home and with peers. Baseline behavioral and school data must be obtained before initiating a trial of medication. Considerations for cultural factors and coexisting psychiatric and physical disorders must be included in the assessment and treatment of patients with ADHD.[30]

Historically, the mainstay treatment for ADHD and US Food and Drug Administration (FDA) –approved medications has been psychostimulants: methylphenidate (methylphenidate), dextroamphetamine, and mixed amphetamine salts. Newer drugs, such as selective noradrenaline reuptake inhibitor, atomoxetine, and 2 selective $\alpha$-adrenergic agonists, extended-release guanfacine and extended-release clonidine, have proven effectiveness in the treatment of core symptoms.[36,37] Clinical concerns associated with prescribing these medications include maintaining a fine line between the therapeutic or efficacy levels and levels related to adverse side effects.[38]

### Psychostimulants

Psychostimulants have been shown to be effective in improving behavior, academic performance, and social adjustment (50% to 95% of children with ADHD).[12] The efficacy of these agents lies in the ability to increase the availability of dopamine, enhancing attention. They also produce a paradoxic calming and mental focusing at low doses and reduction of hyperactive motor movements at higher stimulant doses among patients diagnosed with the disorder as opposed to normal subjects. Another difference is that there is little or no evidence of "reverse tolerance" or sensitization seen in amphetamine or cocaine abusers. Psychostimulants are classified as cognitive enhancers and have been shown to be safe and efficacious in the treatment of school-age children and are considered the drug of choice for the treatment of ADHD. Research indicates that stimulant medications and desipramine improve core symptoms more effectively than placebo and that currently available stimulants have equal efficacy and may improve core ADHD symptoms in 80% of accurately diagnosed children.[39] Part of managing ADHD involves tracking how well the patient responds to the management plan and adjusting therapy, as appropriate, to best suit the needs of the patient.[40]

Although stimulants as a rule have a safe side-effect profile, they can produce adverse side effects. Adverse effects include insomnia, decreased appetite, stomach pain, and headache, and worsening of tics, decreased growth velocity, tachycardia, blood pressure elevation rebound or deterioration when medication wears off, emotional lability, irritability, social withdrawal, and flattened affect.[30] Nursing implications for patients taking stimulants include obtaining an informed consent, providing health education, and gathering baseline information concerning the patient's mental and physical status. Height and weight; diagnostic laboratory studies, including liver enzymes; and vital signs are crucial to monitoring for adverse side effects. In the case of using other drugs that are cardiotoxic, such as desipramine, an electrocardiogram is necessary as baseline and periodic monitoring throughout treatment. Apart from these side effects, in 2009, the FDA issued a black-box warning about atomoxetine and its relationship to increased suicide risks in children and adolescents taking this medication. The agency also stipulated that youth taking this medication must be monitored regularly to assess suicide risk and adherence to medication regimens.

They also need to be seen face to face weekly during the first month of treatment, then every other week for a month, in 12 weeks, and thereafter as clinically indicated. Parents must be educated about symptoms to report to the providers, including a change in behavior (ie, increased agitation) and reports of suicidal ideations and/or behaviors. Similar to stimulants, primary side effects associated with this medication include liver damage and cardiovascular events (ie, sudden death).[12]

Normally, stimulants are ordered on a specified schedule. Stimulant medication is initiated with a low dose and titrated weekly according to patient response and side-effect profile. Beginning with a morning dose enables comparison of morning and afternoon performance. The afternoon dose should be initiated based on severity of symptoms plus time course. After-school dosing enables homework performance without sacrificing sleep latency.[13,14,28] Health education must spell out explicitly benefits and adverse side effects and symptoms that require immediate medical attention. After school dosing is important as well for adolescents who drive, as improved concentration is essential for the inexperienced young driver with ADHD. This also applies to after school activities such as sports, lessons, and work. Information about when to take the medication and monitoring of the patient's appetite and sleeping patterns must be explained to caregivers.

### Nonstimulants

As previously discussed, a new classification of non-stimulant drugs has been approved by the FDA to treat ADHD: atomoxetine and 2 selective α-adrenergic agonists: extended-release guanfacine and extended-release clonidine. The usual process for prescribing all medications is to start low and titrate the dose based on core symptom remission and nominal side effects. Therapeutic response time for these medications ranges from 2 to 8 weeks. In comparison to treatment response to stimulants and nonstimulants, the latter patients are likely to exhibit a slower response. These drugs are less likely to have abuse potential than psychostimulants. Extended release clonidine and extended-release guanfacine are implicated as a monotherapy and as adjunctive therapy to stimulants.[41] Nurses are encouraged to inform parents and caregivers that even though medications may improve academic and social performance, they are not useful in addressing learning disabilities and that other nonpharmacologic approaches, such as psychotherapeutic, behavioral, and psychoeducation, are necessary to help the patient optimize functional, social, and academic performance.

### PSYCHOTHERAPEUTIC INTERVENTIONS

Comprehensive treatment planning must be strength-based and person-centered to meet the needs of the patient, caregivers, and family members. Combined therapies often yield the best results for reduction in symptoms over medication alone, behavioral treatment alone, or community care.[12]

### PSYCHOSOCIAL INTERVENTIONS

Adolescent or adult (best to decrease use of child as the adolescent or adult are often not treated). Psychosocial interventions include helping the child with ADHD gain social skills and more satisfying interactions with peers and family members. Team sports, scouting, and church and community activities are valuable in promoting self-esteem and improving positive relationships with peers and others. Individual therapy and family therapy may be useful, especially for the child with coexisting conditions.[12] These interventions are not a substitute for medication management. It is essential for the parents to comprehend fully the biologic nature of the disorder and the importance of medication adherence to help the child. The ADHD adult may require counseling about his or her condition, vocational assessment and counseling to find the most suitable work environment, time management and organizational assistance, and other suggestions for coping with the disorder. Spouses may benefit from learning about the disorder as well.[21]

Nurses provide an array of psychotherapeutic interventions. Depending on the nurse's educational preparation and clinical expertise, the nurse is likely to play key roles in health education, prescribing medications and/or monitoring the effects of medications, crisis intervention, and providing individual, group-based parenting classes that assist the patient and family in improving coping, parenting, and social skills.

## BEHAVIORAL INTERVENTIONS AND PSYCHOEDUCATION

Behavioral interventions are used to identify and provide positive reinforcement of adaptive coping behaviors to reduce problem behaviors. They are most effective when parents and teachers focus on a limited number of specific behaviors and the environmental conditions that elicit them.[12,30] Effective parental management strategies for parenting the ADHD child have been promulgated by Barkley[13,14] and supported by parent support associations, such as Children and Adults with Attention Deficit Disorders and Attention Deficit Disorder Association. Suggested strategies that promote parental management of difficult behaviors include the following:

1. Give the child more immediate feedback and consequences: positive feedback is given promptly with verbal praise, and negative feedback and consequences are given with specifics as to what the child has done wrong.
2. Give the child frequent feedback (eg, for staying on task during homework).
3. Use larger and more powerful consequences to develop and maintain positive behaviors.
4. Use incentives before punishment.
5. Strive for consistency—being consistent overtime, not giving up too soon, being consistent in various settings, maintaining a united parental front.
6. Act; do not talk.
7. Plan ahead for problem situations by doing the following: stop before entering a problem situation, review the rules in that situation, and ask the child to repeat the rules, set up the reward or incentive, explain the punishment, and follow the plan.
8. Keep a disability perspective.
9. Do not personalize the problems or disorder.
10. Practice forgiveness—let go of bitterness over the child's difficult behavior, forgive others, and forgive yourself.[13,14]
11. Goal-setting in ADHD goes beyond improving symptoms, and should establish observable, measurable targets meaningful to the individual and significant others.

It is imperative for the nurse to develop an individualized psychoeducational program for parents, caregivers, and family members about the disorder of ADHD to understand and have reasonable and realistic expectations. Other management strategies include establishing house rules, routines, and schedules; being specific about behavioral expectations; scheduling time with the child; making frequent eye contact during communication with the child; focusing on the child's strengths; and picking battles carefully. The daily school report card is an educational and behavioral intervention for helping the ADHD child. Examples of daily report cards are found in the Barkley manual.[13,14] The advantage of these report cards include giving the child immediate feedback, helping the parent see trends and changes in behavior, and determining rewards and consequences.

### Group-Based and Parenting Classes

Family therapy and parental training are also indicated in the treatment of ADHD. According to practice guidelines for ADHD, group-based parenting psychoeducation are the first-line treatment for parents and caregivers.[28] Growing evidence suggests that while parenting training may improve parental mental health and parenting skills, it seems to have little or short-term impact on ADHD symptoms and behaviors that impact social and academic performance beyond the home.[42–44] Parents may benefit from learning negotiation, problem solving, and contingency contracting. When the family system is disorganized or chaotic, it is essential for the psychiatric mental health nurse to involve the family and parents in family therapy and parenting classes. Treatment of psychiatric disorders in the parents may be helpful.[12]

### CLASS-BASED BEHAVIORAL INTERVENTIONS

Academic interventions may maximize the likelihood of the child's academic success by developing areas of strength, adapting to special needs, and remediating knowledge and skill deficits. Schools are legally responsible for determining whether the child can meet criteria for special services, such as tutoring or adaptation of educational methods, and ensuring that these services are provided. The Individuals with Disabilities Education Act and Section 504 of the Rehabilitation Act of 1973 provide coverage for children with ADHD. When the disability adversely affects educational performance, eligibility for special education should be approached through the Individuals with Disabilities Education Act. When the disability does not affect educational performance but limits one or more major life activities, eligibility is through Section 504.

Most experts recognize that teachers play an important role in assisting the child with ADHD to succeed. International recommendations[28] suggest that teachers complete training about ADHD and management to help youths with ADHD. It is essential for parents and teachers to work closely together. Daily report cards are an example of this type of close communication and cooperation. The effectiveness of the report card program depends on the teacher accurately evaluating the child's behavior and the consistent use of fair and consistent consequences at home. Children are not adequate or appropriate self-reporters of behavior at school. Missing or absent report cards should be treated the same as a "bad" report. The teacher rates the children using a 5-point system (1 $\frac{1}{4}$ excellent; 2 $\frac{1}{4}$ good; 3 $\frac{1}{4}$ fair; 4 $\frac{1}{4}$ poor; 5 $\frac{1}{4}$ very poor). Teachers are encouraged to write a brief summary for particularly negative behavior.[12]

### SUMMARY

ADHD is a complex neurodevelopmental disorder that exists in children, adolescents, and adults. It places tremendous burden on individuals, families, and communities. This lifelong disorder challenges nurses in various practice settings to understand the basis of ADHD, analyze symptoms, differentiate coexisting disorders, gather health information from varied sources, and implement person-centered multimodal treatment. Nurses are poised to plan and work with patients, families, and teachers in the community and school systems to optimize academic and occupational performance and improve quality of life. Pharmacotherapy, psychoeducation, and behavioral therapies are strong components of multimodal treatment planning.

## REFERENCES

1. American Psychiatric Association:Diagnostic and Statistical Manual of Mental Disorders, Fifth Edition, Arlington (VA): American Psychiatric Association; 2013.
2. Willcutt EG. The prevalence of DSM-IV attention-deficit/hyperactivity disorder: a meta-analytic review. Neurotherapeutics 2012;9:490–9.
3. Polanczyk G, de Lima MS, Horta BL, et al. The worldwide prevalence of ADHD: a systematic review and metaregression analysis. Am J Psychiatry 2007;164:942–8.
4. Simon V, Czobor P, Bálint S, et al. Prevalence and correlates of adult attention-deficit hyperactivity disorder: a meta-analysis. Br J Psychiatry 2009;194:204–11.
5. Antonucci D, Behavioral Health Care Therapist Educational Guide. Available at: www.adhdsharedfocus.com.
6. Collins KP, Cleary SD. Racial and ethnic disparities in parent reported diagnosis of ADHD: National Survey of Children's Health (2003, 2007 and 2011). J Clin Psychiatry 2016;77(1):52–9.
7. American Psychiatric Association. Diagnostic and statistical manual of mental disorders. 5th edition. Washington, DC: Author; 2013.
8. Shaw P, Malek M, Watson B, et al. Trajectories of cerebral cortical development in childhood and adolescence and adult attention-deficit/hyperactivity disorder. Biol Psychiatry 2013;74(8):599–606.
9. Pingault J-B, Viding E, Galera C, et al. Genetic and environmental influences on the developmental course of attention-deficit/hyperactivity disorder symptoms from childhood to adolescence. JAMA Psychiatry 2015;72:651–8.
10. Akutagava-Martins GC, Rohde LA, Hutz MH. Genetics of attention-deficit/hyperactivity disorder: an update. Expert Rev Neurother 2016;16(2):145–56.
11. Cuffe SP, Visser SN, Holbrook JR, et al. ADHD and psychiatric comorbidity: functional outcomes in a school-based sample of children. J Atten Disord 2015. [Epub ahead of print].
12. American Academy of Pediatrics. ADHD: clinical practice guidelines for the diagnosis, evaluation and treatment of attention-deficit/hyperactivity disorder in children and adolescents. Pediatrics 2011;128:1007–22.
13. Barkley RA. Taking charge of ADHD: the complete, authoritative guide for parents. New York: Guilford Press; 2013.
14. Barkley R. Attention-deficit hyperactivity disorder: a handbook for diagnosis and treatment. 3rd edition. New York: Guilford Press; 2006.
15. Bralten J, Franke B, Waldman I, et al. Candidate genetic pathways for attention deficit/hyperactivity disorder (ADHD) show association to hyperactive/impulsive symptoms in children with ADHD. J Am Acad Child Adolesc Psychiatry 2013;52:1204–12.
16. Larsson H, Asherson P, Chang Z, et al. Genetic and environmental influences on adult attention deficit hyperactivity disorder symptoms: a large Swedish population-based study of twins. Psychol Med 2013;43:197–207.
17. Ebejer JL, Medland SE, van der Werf J, et al. Contrast effects and sex influence maternal and self-report dimensional measures of attention-deficit hyperactivity disorder. Behav Genet 2014;45:35–50.

18. Zhou R, Han X, Wang J, et al. Baicalin may have a therapeutic effect in attention deficit hyperactivity disorder. Med Hypotheses 2015;85(6):761–4.
19. Chandler DJ. Evidence for a specialized role of the locus coeruleus noradrenergic system in cortical circuitries and behavioral operations. Brain Res 2015. http://dx.doi.org/10.1016/j.brainres.2015.11.022.
20. Hart H, Chantiluke K, Cubillo AI, et al. Pattern classification of response inhibition in ADHD: toward the development of neurobiological markers for ADHD. Hum Brain Mapp 2013;35:3083–94.
21. Nikolas MA, Burt SA. Genetic and environmental influences on ADHD symptom dimensions of inattention and hyperactivity: a meta-analysis. J Abnorm Psychol 2010;119:1–17.
22. Atabella L, Zoratto F, Adriani W, et al. MR imaging-detectable metabolic alterations in attention deficit/hyperactivity disorder: from preclinical to clinical studies. AJNR Am J Neuroradiol 2014;35:S55–63.
23. Schweren L, Hartman CA, Heslenfeld DJ, et al. Thinner medial temporal cortex in adolescents with attention-deficit/hyperactivity disorder and the effects of stimulants. J Am Acad Child Adolesc Psychiatry 2015;54:660–7.
24. Bendiksen B, Aase H, Diep LM, et al. The associations between pre- and postnatal maternal symptoms of distress and preschooler's symptoms of ADHD, oppositional defiant disorder, conduct disorder, and anxiety. J Atten Disord 2015. [Epub ahead of print].
25. Aoyama Y, Toriumi K, Mouri A, et al. Prenatal nicotine exposure impairs the proliferation of neuronal progenitors, leading to fewer glutamatergic neurons in the medial prefrontal cortex. Neuropsychopharmacology 2016;41:578–89.
26. Nigg JT, Lewis K, Edinger T, et al. Meta-analysis of attention-deficit/hyperactivity disorder or attention-deficit/hyperactivity disorder symptoms, restriction diet, and synthetic food color additives. J Am Acad Child Adolesc Psychiatry 2012;51: 86–97.
27. Stevens LJ, Kuczek T, Burgess JR, et al. Dietary sensitivities and ADHD symptoms: thirty-five years of research. Clin Pediatr (Phila) 2011;50:279–93.
28. National Institute for Health and Care Excellence (NICE). Attention deficit hyperactivity disorder: diagnosis and management. Manchester (UK): NICE; 2008. p. 1–54.
29. Achenbach TM, Rescorla LA. Manual for the ASEBA school-age forms and profiles. Burlington (VT): University of Vermont, Research Center for Children, Youth, & Families; 2001.
30. Brito GN. The Conners abbreviated teacher rating scale: development of norms in Brazil. J Abnorm Child Psychol 1987;15:511–8.
31. Hovik KT, Plessen KJ, Cavanna AE, et al. Cognition, emotion and behavior in children with Tourette's syndrome and children with ADHD-combined subtype—a two-year follow-up study. PLoS One 2015;10:e0144874.
32. Biederman J, Petty CR, Woodworth KY, et al. Adult outcome of attention-deficit/hyperactivity disorder: a controlled 16-year follow-up study. J Clin Psychiatry 2012;73:941–50.
33. Kessler KT, Green JG, Adler LA, et al. Structure and diagnosis of adult attention-deficit/hyperactivity disorder: analysis of expanded symptom criteria from the Adult ADHD Clinical Diagnostic Scale. Arch Gen Psychiatry 2010;67:1168–78.
34. Jaber L, Kirsh D, Diamond G, et al. Long-term functional outcomes in Israeli adults diagnosed in childhood with attention deficit hyperactivity disorder. Isr Med Assoc J 2015;17:481–5.

35. Hinshaw SP, Arnold LE, For the MTA Cooperative Group. ADHD, multimodal treatment, and longitudinal outcome: evidence, paradox, and challenge. Wiley Interdiscip Rev Cogn Sci 2015;6:39–52.
36. Chronis-Tuscano A, Clarke TL, O'Brien KA, et al. Development and preliminary evaluation of an integrated treatment targeting parenting and depressive symptoms in mothers of children with attention-deficit/hyperactivity disorder. J Consult Clin Psychol 2013;81:918–25.
37. Bolea-Almanac B, Nutt DJ, Adamou M, et al. Evidence-based guidelines for the pharmacological management of attention deficit hyperactivity disorder: update on recommendations from the British Association for Psychopharmacology. J Psychopharmacol 2014;28:179–203.
38. Heal DJ, Smith SL, Findling RL. ADHD: current and future therapeutics. Curr Top Behav Neurosci 2012;9:361–90.
39. Otasowie J, Castells X, Ehimare UP, et al. Tricyclic antidepressants for attention deficit hyperactivity disorder (ADHD) in children and adolescents. Cochrane Database Syst Rev 2014;(9):CD006997.
40. Pliska S. Practice parameter for the assessment and treatment of children and adolescent with attention-deficit/hyperactivity disorder. J Am Aca Child Adolesc Psychiatry 2007;46(7):894–921.
41. Golmirzaei J, Mahboobi H, Yazdanparast M, et al. Psychopharmacology of attention-deficit hyperactivity disorder: effects and side effects. Curr Pharm Des 2016;22(5):590–4.
42. Epstein R, Fonnesbeck C, Williamson E, et al. Psychosocial and pharmacologic interventions for disruptive behavior in children and adolescents: comparative effectiveness reviews, No. 154. Rockville (MD): Agency for Healthcare Research and Quality (US); 2015. Report No: 15(16)-EHC019-EF.
43. Zwi M, Jones H, Thorgaard C, et al. Parent training interventions for attention deficit hyperactivity disorder (ADHD) in children aged 5 to 18 years. Cochrane Database Syst Rev 2011;(7):CD003018.
44. Furlong M, McGilloway S, Bywater T, et al. Cochrane Review: behavioural and cognitive-behavioural group-based parenting programmes for early-onset conduct problems in children aged 3 to 12 years (Review). Evid Based Child Health 2012;8:318–692.

# Nursing Care Considerations for the Hospitalized Patient with an Eating Disorder

Barbara E. Wolfe, PhD, RN, PMHCNS-BC*,
Julie P. Dunne, MSN, RN, PMHNP-BC, Meredith R. Kells, MSN, RN, CPNP

## KEYWORDS

- Anorexia nervosa • Bulimia nervosa • Binge eating disorder • Eating disorders
- Inpatient • Hospitalization • Nursing diagnoses • Nursing care

## KEY POINTS

- Eating disorders are serious conditions.
- A comprehensive nursing assessment is essential.
- Nursing interventions are tailored to the individual needs for optimal outcomes.

Eating disorders are chronic psychiatric illnesses with significant medical complications, psychological distress, and psychiatric comorbidity. In addition to being a public health concern,[1] eating disorders are among those psychiatric illnesses having the highest mortality.[2] Although many patients are treated on an outpatient basis, inpatient care for the more severely ill patient can be challenging given the severity of illness and concurrent issues. This article provides an overview of the clinical characteristics of eating disorders typically seen for inpatient care and key areas for nursing assessment and intervention during hospitalization.

## EPIDEMIOLOGY

Anorexia nervosa (AN) affects 0.3% to 2.2% of women over the lifetime and bulimia nervosa (BN) affects 1% to 3% of this same group.[3] Binge eating disorder (BED) affects up to 3.5%% of the population.[3] The number of men with eating disorders is

This article is an update of an article previously published in Nursing Clinics of North America, Volume 38, Issue 1, March 2003.
Disclosure Statement: The authors have no known commercial or financial conflicts of interest.
Boston College Wm. F. Connell School of Nursing, Maloney Hall, 140 Commonwealth Avenue, Chestnut Hill, MA 02467, USA
* Corresponding author.
E-mail address: wolfeb@bc.edu

increasing in recent years due to changes in diagnostic criteria and reporting; however, overall, women are up to 3 times more likely to be affected.[1] Onset of AN and BN is typically during adolescent and early adulthood but may occur at other ages. BED is more likely to begin later in life.[4] These disorders seem to be most prevalent in Western cultures, although studies suggest that binge eating behavior is equally or more common in minority groups compared with white samples.[5]

## CAUSES

Although the cause of eating disorders is elusive, several factors are likely to have a contributory role. Sociocultural and environmental factors, including the media and peer influences, are thought to be influential.[6] Family characteristics, including parenting styles,[7] dynamics and discord,[8] and parental personalities,[9] likely play a role. Biological variables, including genetics, neurotransmitter regulation, and hormonal functioning, have been implicated.[6] Negative affect, low self-esteem, and dieting commonly predate the onset of an eating disorder, although causality has not been shown. Because none of these factors offers a sufficient explanation alone, it is likely that there are several pathways to the development of an eating disorder, and the possibility of a constellation of interactive factors contributing to vulnerability and expression.

## DIAGNOSTIC CRITERIA
### Anorexia Nervosa

The Diagnostic Statistical Manual of Mental Disorders, 5th edition (DSM-5) defines AN as occurring in individuals who restrict their energy intake resulting in a significantly low body weight or, in the case of children and adolescents "less than minimally expected."[10] These individuals are terrified of gaining weight and are severely influenced by a distorted perception of their own body shape and weight.[10] AN is classified into 2 subtypes: (1) restricting, with no routine binge eating or purging; and (2) binge-eating / purging, with regular binge or purge episodes.[10]

### Bulimia Nervosa

BN occurs in individuals who are in a normal weight range or who may be overweight. Patients experience recurring binge eating episodes characterized by the consumption of a large amount of food in a short period of time accompanied by a loss of control over the behavior. To avoid gaining weight, patients use inappropriate purging (eg, self-induced vomiting, laxative abuse, enemas) or nonpurging (eg, fasting, diuretics, extreme exercise) compensatory behaviors. Frequency of binge eating and compensatory episodes averages at least once a week for 3 months or more.[10] As with AN, body shape and weight are pivotal to self-esteem.

### Other Eating and Feeding Disorders

Several other eating and feeding disorders sometimes are encountered in the hospital setting. BED is characterized by repeated binges, similar to those seen in BN, occurring at least once weekly.[10] Unlike BN, no compensatory behaviors occur in BED; thus, these individuals tend to be above normal weight. Binges cause distress and are often associated with rapid eating and feeling uncomfortably full despite not being physically hungry.[10] More common to infancy and early childhood are pica, rumination disorder, and avoidant / restrictive food intake disorder.[10] "Other specified" and "unspecified" feeding or eating disorders are diagnoses used when individuals do not meet full criteria for 1 of the former diagnoses or there is a need for more information.[10]

## COMORBID DISORDERS

Comorbid psychiatric disorders often occur in patients with AN, BN, and BED. Approximately 70% of affected individuals will have at least 1 other psychiatric diagnoses.[11] The most common co-occurring diagnoses include anxiety disorders, mood disorders, and substance disorders.[11] As many as one-third of patients report engaging in nonsuicidal self-injury during the past year.[12] Hospitalized patients with AN and BN may present with increased aggressive and impulsive behaviors.[13] Trauma history, such as childhood sexual abuse, is associated with BN and BED.[14] Patients with borderline personality disorder have higher rates of BN, whereas those with obsessive-compulsive personality disorder have higher rates of AN.[15] Obsessive-compulsive and avoidant are the most frequent personality disorders seen in BED.[16] Generally, the presence of comorbidities is a predictor of health services utilization among individuals with mental illness.[17]

## PROGNOSIS

Eating disorders are often chronic conditions. A follow-up study of adolescents with AN 4 to 20 years after hospitalization showed outcomes were 68% positive, 23% intermediate, and approximately 9% poor across a range of biopsychosocial indicators.[18] Rate of recovery increases with duration of follow-up time; for example, approximately 33% of individuals at 4 years and 73% at 10 years or more were recovered.[19] The highest risk period for relapse of AN is in the first year following hospitalization or day treatment.[20] In a 5-year follow-up study of BN, rate of remission and relapse was approximately 74% and 47%, respectively.[21] Twenty-year follow-up suggests a 75% remission rate for BN.[22] Long-term rates of recovery from BN range from approximately 40% to 67% in the first 5 and 10 years.[23] High frequency of pretreatment binge eating and vomiting is associated with rapid relapse of BN.[24] Longitudinal studies of BED suggest recovery rates ranging from 50% to 85% following 4 to 6 years.[25]

## INPATIENT NURSING CARE
### Therapeutic Relationship

The relationship between the provider and the patient is vital to inpatient nursing care. The nurse plays a crucial role in creating and fostering a therapeutic alliance. Defining attributes of this alliance include mutual partnership, consumer focus, and consumer empowerment.[26] Empathy, respect, acceptance, compassion, trust, hope, rapport, and the ability to be nonjudgmental are thought to be particularly essential.[26] The therapeutic alliance may be particularly influential for treatment outcomes in AN.[27] Interactions are influenced by several factors, including experiences, attitudes, and perceptions of both the nurse and the patient.

### Nurse

Nurses, as do patients, live in a society often obsessed with food, body size, and dieting. These issues may hold meaning for professionals who are experiencing their own struggles and lead to feelings of shame, ambivalence, and envy when working with patients with idealized body size. This may contribute to overidentification with, and minimization of, the patient's pathologic behavior and cognitions. It can be difficult to imagine why a person would starve herself or himself. The emaciated state of some anorexic patients can be shocking. It can be normal for the nurse to feel perplexed and frustrated because this can challenge the core values of the nurse.[28]

Because patients with eating disorders are typically intellectually bright, engaging, and, with the exception of emaciated states or significant comorbidity, appear otherwise nonimpaired, the severity of their disorder and distress may be underestimated. On busy inpatient units, the needs of patients with eating disorders are at risk for being secondary to others because they erroneously are perceived as less sick. Keeping in mind the significant psychiatric comorbidity, complications, and associated mortality rates, it is crucial that the nurse not be derailed by such misinterpretations because these patients are significantly ill.

### Patient

Hospitalization may evoke feelings in the patient that affects the therapeutic relationship. Medical instability, significant comorbidity, or the influence of a parent, loved one, or therapist often leads to hospitalization. It does not usually happen as a result of patient insight because denial of severity is classic and can contribute to resistance to a therapeutic connection[29] and treatment.[30] Patients who are hospitalized involuntarily may express complete denial of illness and a sense of having no control over the present situation because they already experience little control over most aspects of his or her life. For many, loss of control heightens issues of trust that play a crucial role in the therapeutic relationship.

Treatment goals are often in direct opposition to the patient's desires. Hospitalization heightens fear of weight gain, and for patients with AN, this is exactly what they have been desperately avoiding. Control often is expressed through rigidity, which is likely an attempt to maintain a sense of self-efficacy and order. It is important to be attentive to issues of control because these can lead power struggles between the patient and nurse. Fear and anxiety are common. Feelings of distress or dread frequently compete for the patient's attention while the provider earnestly tries to engage them. This can represent a significant barrier to communication. The eating disorder may be an identity for the person and the thought of no longer having it may contribute to a sense of overwhelming trepidation.[31]

## NURSING PLAN OF CARE
### Key Areas of Assessment

A comprehensive assessment includes evaluation of chief complaint, mental status, and social, developmental, family, medical, and psychiatric treatment history. Evaluation of coping mechanisms, resources, and social support should occur. Key areas pertinent to the assessment of the patient with an eating disorder are discussed in more detail.

### Chief Complaint

The patient's chief complaint and reason for hospitalization provide information regarding insight, primary concerns, treatment adherence issues, and motivation. Motivation to recover predicts treatment outcomes and those less motivated are more likely to leave treatment prematurely.[32]

### Mental Status

A mental status examination is indicated on admission. In addition to the standard areas, particular attention to mood and affect is warranted, given the high rates of comorbidity. A thorough assessment of suicidal ideation, plans, and attempts is indicated. Psychomotor function, appearance, and speech also may provide information about the presence of depressive symptoms. Judgment, reliability, and insight are likely to be more impaired during an acute stage of illness.

### Developmental and Social History

Developmental milestones (eg, individuation, separation, identity) and social history (eg, academic progress, occupation, peer relations, traumatic events, drug or alcohol use) plotted on a timeline can be informative when assessing the relationship of events with symptoms. Patients often describe social influences affecting their desire to change body shape or weight, such as childhood teasing about weight or weight restrictions of extracurricular activities such as crew, ballet, gymnastics, cheerleading, and wrestling. The time spent preoccupied with body shape and weight, and on compensatory behaviors, can leave these individuals socially isolated. Individuals with a high degree of drive for thinness, body dissatisfaction, and bulimic symptoms may avoid eating with others because of social anxiety and fear of being evaluated negatively.[33]

Alcohol and drug use often start in a social context. Because of the prevalence of comorbid substance abuse, review of alcohol and drug use is necessary (eg, amount, frequency, and duration). Some drugs (eg, stimulants, caffeine, diet pills) may be abused because of their effects on metabolism and weight loss. Patients with BN may report binge drinking. Blackouts and loss of consciousness should be noted.

### Family History and Functioning

The family is an important source of information for understanding its potential influence on the patient and the meaning of the disorder. Family norms related to eating, perceptions of body weight and shape, cultural values, history of obesity or eating disorders, and other psychopathology are areas to explore. Assessing the history and relationships among family members on a genogram provides data on conflictual, distant, vulnerable, harmonic, and triangulated relations.[34] Plotting family events on a timeline (eg, births, deaths, divorces) provides an opportunity to assess the relationship with onset or severity of eating-related symptoms.

### Medical History and Current Medical Problems

A medical history, in addition to information obtained from a physical examination, is important to assess (1) previous illnesses, (2) medical complications and degree of malnutrition secondary to the eating disorder, and (3) other potential medical and psychiatric conditions that may be the underlying cause of symptoms. Medical complications of an eating disorder are many and are summarized in **Table 1**. Differential diagnoses that may mimic some symptoms of the eating disorder are presented in **Table 2**.

### Psychiatric Treatment History

Psychiatric treatment history includes current and past outpatient therapies, participation in residential and day programs, and hospitalizations. Date, duration, therapist, location, diagnosis, treatment modality, and response are noted. History of pharmacologic intervention is useful (eg, medication name, dose, duration, response, and efficacy). Use, benefit, and adherence to adjunct therapies, including nutritional counseling, group therapies, and support groups, provide information on available resources, barriers, and utilization of various modes of intervention.

### Eating Patterns and Compensatory Behaviors

Assessment of eating patterns includes frequency, type, and location of food intake. Many patients with AN report limiting themselves to less than 1000 kcal per day.[38] This limitation is significant because daily caloric needs for young women are 2000 to

**Table 1**
**Medical complications**

| System | Signs and Symptoms |
|---|---|
| Cardiovascular | Bradycardia (<60 beats per minute), hypotension (<90/60 mm Hg), orthostatic hypotension, cardiac palpitations and arrhythmias (associated with hypokalemia), electrocardiogram abnormalities (nonspecific S-T wave changes, prolonged Q-Tc interval, U waves [in the presence of hypokalemia and hypomagnesemia]), cardiomyopathy (associated with emetine toxicity from abuse of syrup of ipecac), persistent junctional rhythm, left ventricular atrophy, mitral valve prolapse, pericardial effusions<br>AN: congestive heart failure (rare; associated with rapid refeeding), sudden death (rare; associated with prolonged Q-T interval and arrhythmia) |
| Dermatologic | Abrasions on the knuckles (Russell's sign; related to self-induced vomiting), xerosis, acrocyanosis, carotenoderma<br>AN: brittle hair and nails, loss of hair (related to malnutrition), lanugo, loss of subcutaneous fat |
| Endocrine and metabolism | Oligomenorrhea, hypoglycemia, enlarged parotid glands, hyperamylasemia; increased aldosterone, decreased estrogen, luteinizing hormone, follicle-stimulating hormone, testosterone (men)<br>AN: hypothermia, cold intolerance; increased growth hormone, cortisol, cholesterol, and liver function tests; decreased prealbumin; amenorrhea |
| Fluid and electrolytes | Dehydration, elevated blood urea nitrogen, hypokalemia, hypomagnesemia, hyponatremia, hypophosphatemia, metabolic alkalosis (elevated sodium bicarbonate; related to vomiting), metabolic acidosis (reduced sodium bicarbonate; related to laxative abuse)<br>AN: peripheral edema (with refeeding) |
| Gastrointestinal | Constipation, diarrhea (related to laxative abuse), bloating, gastric distention, abdominal cramps, reflux, dysphagia, dyspepsia, hematemesis, irritable bowel syndrome, cathartic colon syndrome (related to laxative abuse), gastric rupture (rare), esophagitis (related to self-induced vomiting), Mallory-Weiss syndrome (esophageal tear; rare), mucositis, dental carries, enamel erosion (related to self-induced vomiting), sensitive teeth<br>AN: delayed gastric emptying, superior mesenteric artery syndrome (related to weight loss) |
| Hematology | Bone marrow suppression (related to phenolphthalein-containing laxatives), anemia<br>AN: leukopenia, neutropenia, thrombocytopenia, decreased albumin |
| Musculoskeletal | AN: fractures, osteopenia, osteoporosis |
| Neurologic | Fatigue, depression, vertigo, syncope<br>AN: pontine myelinolysis (rare); brain atrophy (reversible with weight restoration) |
| Pulmonary | AN: pulmonary edema (rare; associated with rapid refeeding) |

*Abbreviation:* AN, specific to anorexia nervosa.
*Data from* Refs.[35-37]

2400 kcal.[39] Persons with BN often have cycles of restricting intake between binges.[40] Individuals who binge are often reluctant to disclose the amount consumed. Persons with BED tend to eat more meals per day, and have fewer episodes of fasting compared with individuals with BN or AN.[40]

Information about binges is useful (eg, frequency, duration, associated feelings, and events). Typically, these occur in secret and frequency is variable, ranging from a

| Table 2 |  |
|---|---|
| Differential diagnoses for eating disorder symptoms |  |
| Symptom | Differential Diagnoses |
| Weight loss | Depression, alcohol abuse or dependence, substance abuse or dependence (eg, stimulants), peptic ulcer disease, hyperthyroidism, celiac disease, adrenocortical insufficiency, acquired immunodeficiency syndrome, cancer |
| Uncontrollable or increased eating | Prader-Willi syndrome, Kleine-Levin syndrome |
| Preoccupation with body shape | Body dysmorphic disorder |

couple of times per week to several times per day. Binges are composed of foods high in fat and carbohydrates and that are easy to ingest and purge. Caloric binge intake typically ranges from 1200 to 4500 kcal[41] but can be more. Binges place the individual at risk for weight gain and some individuals resort to inappropriate behaviors to compensate.

Assessment of compensatory behaviors, more common in AN and BN, includes type and frequency. Although these patients typically engage in several methods, self-induced vomiting is the most common. Some individuals use mechanical stimulation of the uvula whereas others turn to the use of syrup of ipecac. In cases of the latter, or for individuals who use diuretics, diet pills, and laxatives, quantity is important and often increases over time. Tapering of laxatives may be necessary. Daily exercise also should be reviewed for excessiveness. Some patients may report compulsive exercising for 3 to 4 hours per day to expend calories; this exceeds daily and weekly recommendations for children and adults.[42] Fasting, particularly in patients with AN, can endure for several days at a time. Other means of compensatory behaviors occur and patients should be asked what they do to prevent weight gain.

### Other Core Eating Disorder Symptoms

#### Self-esteem, body image, and cognitive disturbances
Individuals with AN, BN, and BED experience reduced self-esteem[43,44] and body image disturbance,[45,46] contributing to negative self-evaluation and eating disorder symptoms.[47] After a binge, patients typically experience negative mood, shame, and self-disgust.[41] Self-esteem may be influenced by other factors, including comorbidities, perceived failures, and other stressors. Anorexic and bulimic patients have a magnified sense of their own body shape, and this may manifest in complaints about size or shape of stomach, thighs, and buttocks. In BED, overevaluation of body shape and weight is associated with poorer psychosocial functioning.[48]

Patients exhibit cognitive distortions relative to their belief system around food and weight. For AN and BN, foods typically are classified into either "good" or "bad," reflecting dichotomous thinking. Attitudes toward the bad foods may reflect a phobic or illogical response. Magical thinking may occur—including the belief that if one eats a particular food, it immediately will result in fat deposits. Such distortions are evident in the worshiping of thinness despite consequences.

#### Body weight
History of body weight is useful for assessing past eating disorder or obesity. Obtaining highest and lowest weight and fluctuations over time indicate the possibility and severity of compensatory behavior used. For children and adolescents, weight should be assessed using a growth chart (eg, www.cdc.gov/growthcharts).[49] For adults,

relative body weight is typically expressed as body mass index (BMI), calculated as weight (kg) divided by the square height (m²).

### Menstrual cycle

Onset of menses, regularity, and use of hormones (eg, oral contraceptives) to induce menstruation are assessed. Secondary amenorrhea is common to persons with AN. However, dieting behavior, caloric intake, BMI, and exercise have been shown to be associated with secondary amenorrhea and oligomenorrhea in women regardless of eating disorder diagnoses.[50] Assessment of sexual activities, including method of birth control, is indicated.

### Nursing Diagnoses, Desired Outcomes, Goals, and Interventions

Because clinical presentation can be varied, many nursing diagnoses and desired outcomes may be relevant to the care of patients with eating disorders (**Table 3**). Nursing interventions are determined based on the patient's needs, goals, and overall interdisciplinary treatment plan.

### Aims of Hospitalization

Hospitalization typically occurs with patients who are severely medically unstable, suicidal, at a significantly low body weight, in need of structured environment to manage symptoms, and/or experiencing significant acute co-occurring disorders or medical complications.[54,55] Aims of hospitalization are driven by presenting condition and diagnoses and may include weight restoration, treatment of physical complications, restoration of healthy eating patterns, enhanced motivation, nutritional education, improved functioning, treatment of comorbidity, family support, and relapse prevention.[54] Individualized treatment planning and delivery encompasses an interdisciplinary approach.[56]

### Targeted Interventions

Examples of possible nursing interventions are presented in **Table 4**. Additional key areas of consideration are discussed in greater detail here.

### Cognitive disturbances

Cognitive-behavioral techniques are used to address altered perceptions. These strategies are introduced after initial stabilization. Tactics include exploring belief systems, particular tasks (eg, list positive self-attributes), exploring alternative adaptive behaviors; self-monitoring (diaries), and restructuring beliefs, attitudes, and misperceptions. Interventions target incremental change, allowing realistic success. In addition, encouraging attendance at therapy sessions assists in improving cognitive functioning.

### Nutritional requirements, meal patterns, and body weight

For patients with AN, target weight needs to be established collectively. The goal weight is often the weight at which menstruation (for women) or testicular function (for men) is restored.[54] For adolescent, the goal weight is determined by BMI percentile.[57] Generally, a safe rate of weight gain during hospitalization is approximately 2 to 3 pounds per week.[54] Food intake ranges from 30 to 40 kcal/kg/d and is increased up to 70 to 100 kcal/kg/d.[54] This means starting at 1000 to 1600 kcal/d and incrementally increasing to as much as 2100 to 4000 kcal/d. However, some patients with severe food restriction are at risk for refeeding syndrome or are resistant to food intake, and may need to start at a more modest increase.[54,58] Caloric intake is adjusted according to weight gain and maintenance. Weight restoration rate[59] and level[60] have

**Table 3**
Examples of nursing diagnoses related to the care of patients with eating disorders

| Domain Areas & Nursing Diagnoses[a] | Related Factors[a] | Defining Characteristics | Desired Outcome |
|---|---|---|---|
| **Activity or Rest** | | | |
| Cardiac output, decreased; risk for | Alterations heart rate, rhythm, and preload | Bradycardia, electrocardiogram changes, palpitations, fatigue | Adequate cardiac output as evidenced by normal pulse rate, blood pressure, and rhythm |
| **Comfort** | | | |
| Pain, acute | Abdominal cramping, irritation of epigastric and gastric mucosa, gastric distention | Verbal reports, facial grimacing, autonomic response (sudden or severe pain) | Verbalize pain relief using self-report rating scale, follow prescribed pharmacologic regimen, verbalize methods that provide relief, identify and exhibit strategies to prevent recurrence |
| **Coping or Stress Tolerance** | | | |
| Anxiety | Perceived threat to physical body, body image, and self-concept | Expressed concern, apprehension, fear, anguish, distress; preoccupation with body shape and weight; compulsive and ritualistic behavior; difficulty concentrating; decreased ability to problem-solve; autonomic response; nonverbal cues (eg, facial tension, psychomotor agitation) | Reduce anxiety as evidenced by appearance and self-report, acknowledge and discusses fears, recognize healthy and unhealthy fears, identify signs and symptoms of anxiety, identify and demonstrate techniques to decrease anxiety |
| Coping, ineffective | Anxiety, depression, maladaptive response patterns, inadequate social support, maturational crisis | Verbalized inability to cope or request help, impaired cognition and perceptions, diminished problem-solving capacity, use of maladaptive and self-destructive behaviors (eg, verbal manipulation, binge episodes, laxative abuse) | Identify ineffective coping behaviors and consequences, identify and use alternative coping strategies, demonstrate adaptive problem-solving skills, identify crisis prevention resources |
| Coping, family disabled | Ambivalent relations, discordant coping styles, resistance to treatment, and unexpressed feelings among family members | Denial of existence or severity of patient's condition; intolerance, neglect, rejection, hostility, abandonment, enmeshment; overly fixated on patient or patient's illness | Appropriately and openly express feelings; verbalize realistic understanding and expectations of the patient; visit or contact patient regularly; participate positively in the care of the patient within limits of family's ability, patient needs, and treatment plan |

(continued on next page)

**Table 3**
*(continued)*

| Domain Areas & Nursing Diagnoses[a] | Related Factors[a] | Defining Characteristics | Desired Outcome |
|---|---|---|---|
| Denial, ineffective | Inability or refusal to accept presence or severity of illness | Failure to acknowledge symptoms severity, and impact on well-being; minimization of symptoms; seems indifferent when relaying severe signs and symptoms; delay or refusal in seeking treatment; dismissive comments when discussing illness | Increase insight and motivation, exhibit understanding of disease process and prognosis; accept appropriate medical and psychiatric interventions |
| Mood regulation, impaired | Anxiety, depression, psychiatric impairment, weight change | Rapid or prolonged shifts in extreme mood states; observed labile affect; emotional reactivity; social isolation; psychological inflexibility; dysphoria; anger; hostility; irritability; speech may be slow or fast, soft or loud, restricted or expansive, or pressured | Establish coping strategies to deal with challenging emotions and distorted cognitions; manage anxiety, depression, and other symptoms of impaired mood regulation; improve mood regulation and distress tolerance |
| Powerlessness | Hospitalization, treatment plan (eg, weight gain), feelings of helplessness) | Expressed apathy, passivity, uncertainty, or lack of control over therapy or self-care; verbalized dissatisfaction or frustration with limits placed on maladaptive behaviors (eg, self-induced vomiting); inability to stop binge episodes; nonparticipation in care, dependence on others | State sense of control over the present situation and future outcomes, participate in decision-making with regard to plan of care, identify areas within patient's control and those that are not |
| Elimination & Exchange | | | |
| Constipation, risk for | Decreased gastric emptying, poor eating habits and dehydration | Decreased stool frequency; dry, hard, formed stools; straining with defecation; decreased bowel sounds; abdominal or back pain; palpable abdominal mass | Establish normal bowel elimination pattern (soft formed stool q1-3 d), identify contributing factors and appropriate preventative strategies, exhibit adequate fluid and food intake, express relief from associated discomfort |

**Health Promotion**

| | | |
|---|---|---|
| Noncompliance | Value system, health beliefs, cultural factors, motivation, and readiness for change incongruent with plan of care; difficulties in patient-provider relationships | Resistant behavior; nonadherence to treatment regimen; lack of progress and/or failure to meet outcomes; minimization of severity of illness; devaluation of treatment team, plan, and usefulness of therapy; symptom exacerbation and development of associated complications | Participate in the development of treatment goals and plan, demonstrate understanding of disorder and treatment regimen, describe daily nutritional and activity patterns to achieve therapeutic goals, identify consequences of noncompliance |

**Nutrition**

| | | | |
|---|---|---|---|
| Nutrition, imbalanced: less than body requirements | Insufficient dietary intake due to self-imposed severe caloric restriction or refusal to eat, decreased ingestion of food or nutrient absorption secondary to self-induced vomiting and laxative abuse | Food intake below recommended daily allowance, body weight >15% below ideal (may be normal or overweight in BN), weight loss, impaired hunger and satiety, reduced muscle tone and subcutaneous fat, laboratory findings of protein and vitamin deficiencies | Establish regular meal pattern and normal caloric intake to support and maintain normal body weight; show progressive gain toward goal weight; display normalization of laboratory values; free of signs of malnutrition; express understanding of nutritional needs; show adequate food intake, abstinence from binge eating, and use of inappropriate compensatory behaviors |
| Obesity; overweight, risk for | Food intake excessive relative to metabolic need | In adults, BMI 25–29.9 (overweight), >30 (obese); less than recommended daily physical activity; weight gain; report of binge eating episodes; observed dysfunctional eating patterns | Verbalize understanding of nutritional needs and risk for weight gain, show appropriate behavioral change in eating patterns, identify alternative coping strategies rather than binge eating, exhibit abstinence from binge eating |
| Electrolyte imbalance, risk for | Excessive fluid volume, insufficient fluid volume, self-induced vomiting, diarrhea (laxative abuse) | Risk factors: restriction of fluid intake, water-loading, self-induced vomiting, laxative use, abnormal electrolyte laboratory values and associated complications (ie, cardiac abnormalities, edema, altered mental status) | Maintain normal laboratory electrolyte values, stabilize fluid volume, abstinence from vomiting, acknowledge importance of electrolytes to functioning, verbalize causative factors and signs and symptoms of imbalance |

(continued on next page)

**Table 3**
*(continued)*

| Domain Areas & Nursing Diagnoses[a] | Related Factors[a] | Defining Characteristics | Desired Outcome |
|---|---|---|---|
| Fluid volume, deficient, risk for | Loss of fluid through inadequate intake, self-induced vomiting, abuse of laxatives, enemas and/or diuretics | Risk factors: decreased urine output, concentrated urine, output exceeds intake, sudden weight loss, increased serum hematocrit, increased pulse, decreased blood pressure, orthostatic hypotension, weakness, dry skin and poor turgor | Maintain fluid volume at a functional level as evidenced by adequate daily fluid intake, normal vital signs, moist mucous membranes, and good skin turgor; verbalize understanding of causative factors and preventative strategies; demonstrate behaviors promoting adequate hydration |
| Fluid volume, excess; risk for imbalanced fluid volume | Excess fluid related to refeeding | Severe malnutrition requiring the need for refeeding, intentional water-loading to increase weight, abnormal physical findings (eg, low specific gravity, sudden weight gain, edema, electrolyte imbalance) | Maintain normal urine output (minimum of 0.5 mL/kg/h),[51] normal vital signs, and absence of edema; describe understanding of dietary or fluid restrictions; list signs that require further evaluation and notification of care provider |
| **Perception or Cognition** | | | |
| Deficient knowledge regarding condition, prognosis, and/or treatment needs | Inadequate understanding, lack of knowledge, cognitive distortions | Verbalized deficit, inadequate food and fluid intake and development of preventable complications, inadequate follow-through of instructions, misconception of weight loss through use of inappropriate compensatory behaviors | Participate in learning process; explain nutritional, psychological, medical, and social consequences of disorder; exhibit understanding of treatment regimen; verbalize after-care plans including providers, contact information, and appointments; list available resources following discharge |
| **Safety or Protection** | | | |
| Suicide, risk for | Impulsivity, comorbid major depression | Risk factors: history of previous suicide attempts; major depressive episodes; clinically significant depressed mood; suicidal ideation, plan, gesture, or recent attempt; verbalization of feeling sad, blue, hopeless, life is not worth living | Remain safe and harm-free, verbally express feelings, readily discuss suicidal ideation and seeks help, remains free from access to harmful objects, independently maintains self-control |

| | | |
|---|---|---|
| Self-mutilation, risk for | Comorbid borderline personality disorder, dissociation, use of suicidal gestures to manipulate others, inappropriate means to release tension | Risk factors: history of self-injury (eg, cutting, burning, head banging, and/or punching or pinching); history of suicide attempts, impulsivity, or abuse; psychomotor agitation; inability to control anger; inability to verbalize feelings | Remains safe and harm-free, verbally express feelings, readily discuss urge to self-mutilate and seek help, identify precipitating events, engage in use of adaptive coping to manage urges, independently maintains self-control |
| Trauma, risk for | Loss of bone integrity | Risk factors: long-term malnutrition, history of bone fractures or bone loss | Remain trauma-free, demonstrate appropriate behaviors aimed at reducing risk of injury |
| Dentition, impaired | Chronic self-induced vomiting | Enamel discoloration or erosion, dental pain | Verbalize understanding of appropriate oral hygiene, access dental care, abstinence from vomiting |
| Self-Perception | | | |
| Body image, disturbed | Cognitive distortions of actual body size, shape, and/or appearance | Negative feelings or expression of shame and guilt about body shape and/or weight, concealment of body with oversized clothing, depends on other's opinions regarding body weight and/or shape | Improve or normalize perception of size, shape, and/or appearance; verbalize congruence between self-perceived and actual body shape and/or size; state positive aspects about body |
| Self-esteem, situational low | Negative self-evaluation | Negative self-worth, expressed shame or guilt, rejection of positive feedback, dwells on negative feedback, indecisive; seeks reassurance repeatedly, dependent, self-value solely determined by body shape and weight | Demonstrate behaviors aimed at promoting positive self-esteem, verbalize increased sense of self-esteem and self-acceptance, verbalize personal strengths |

For additional resources see Ackley & Ladwig,[51] Herdman & Kamisturu,[52] and Townsend.[53]
a Based on NANDA-I (formerly known as North American Nursing Diagnosis Association) Taxonomy and Domains.[52]

**Table 4**
Nursing diagnoses and examples of related interventions for the nursing care of hospitalized patients eating disorders

| Nursing Diagnoses | Potential Interventions (Determined by the Individual Case) |
|---|---|
| Anxiety | Assist to identify perceived threats; assess level of anxiety and physical response, listen and encourage to express feelings, acknowledge patient's fears, assist to identify antecedents as well as signs and symptoms of anxiety, assess coping mechanism used to relieve anxiety, reinforce positive coping skills and teach additional options (eg, relaxation techniques), develop plan to try alternative measures for relief of anxiety, provide positive reinforcement and feedback for use of adaptive measures, administer antianxiety agents as ordered and monitor for therapeutic and adverse effects |
| Body image, disturbed | Assess body perception, impact on functioning, and family and social influences contributing to disturbance; determine extent to which patient's body image is congruent with reality (eg, have the patient draw self on wall with chalk, then compare with actual body outline); allow for expression of fears; assist to correct distortions through use of journal of thoughts, feelings, and assumptions related to body image; provide positive feedback as appropriate and refuting evidence for distorted beliefs; explore positive aspects of body |
| Cardiac output, decreased, risk for | Review and monitor laboratory findings (eg, complete blood count, electrolytes, blood urea nitrogen) and report abnormal values to primary clinician, monitor vital signs, review diagnostic studies (eg, electrocardiogram), monitor fluid input and output, restrict fluids as ordered, explain dietary restrictions (eg, low sodium), elevate feet if edema present, educate about positional changes to avoid orthostatic hypotension and about signs of improved cardiac output (eg, reduced peripheral edema, improved vital signs or blood pressures) |
| Constipation, risk for | Assess contributing factors, including medication; discuss usual elimination patterns and initiate regular schedule; use diary for self-monitoring of frequency, time of day, and characteristics of stool; encourage adequate daily fluid and fiber intake as appropriate for age, gender, and physiologic factors[39], assess for pain; palpate abdomen for distention and masses; auscultate abdomen for bowel sounds; palpate abdomen for distention and masses; administer gastrointestinal agents as ordered; educate about role of diet and fluid intake on normal bowel function; assist in creating a plan if problem reoccurs |
| Coping, ineffective | Assess insight and motivation for change, impact of illness, risk for suicide, and previous use, effect, and types of coping; explore fears, sense of control, and meaning of illness; assist to identify needs that are being met with sick role; address manipulation directly and openly; use food diary to self-monitor factors precipitating urge to binge and engage in compensatory behaviors; identify list of at-risk situations vulnerable to ineffective coping; use role playing to teach and model problem-solving skills; teach alternative coping strategies (eg, mindfulness, assertiveness techniques); provide positive feedback and build in self-reward for successful coping (eg, abstinence from self-induced vomiting) |
| Coping, family disabled | Establish rapport with available family members; maintain effective communication; meet to assess contributing factors to disabled coping and identify strengths; explore impact, perceptions, and meaning of patient's illness; encourage questions, expression of feelings and concerns, and participation in therapeutic activities (eg, family therapy, groups, visits); provide reality-based information to address unrealistic expectations and perceptions of severity of illness; help to establish appropriate boundaries between family members; assist to reframe negative comments or criticism; provide appropriate referral and information on additional resources (see **Table 5**) |

| | |
|---|---|
| Denial, ineffective | Establish rapport and build toward trusting relationship; assist in identifying impact of disease on life, and explore current perceptions of symptoms and needs; increase insight and motivation (eg, verbalize and explore feelings related to fear of gaining weight); assist to explore alternative ways to feel in control within environment (eg, make a list of pros and cons of treatment); explore fears associated with treatment; provide reality testing |
| Dentition, impaired | Promote routine biannual dental assessments, cleanings, and additional dental care as needed; encourage adequate oral hygiene as indicated (eg, flossing daily, brushing with fluoride-containing toothpaste, using soft bristles); encourage cessation of purging behaviors and maintenance of appropriate nutrition and fluid intake |
| Electrolyte imbalance, risk for | Be aware of signs and symptoms of electrolyte imbalances (eg, muscle twitches, palpitations); assess gastric, cardiac, and neurologic functioning, as well as pain level and mental status; monitor laboratory values (eg, serum electrolytes, pH, comprehensive metabolic panel, blood gases); vital signs, including cardiac rhythm, and fluid intake and output, and report abnormalities to primary clinician; teach patient the importance of stable electrolyte values for healthy functioning |
| Fluid volume, deficient, risk for | Monitor fluid intake and output and fluctuations in daily weight (AN); encourage adequate daily fluid intake as appropriate for age, gender, and physiologic factors[39]; assess mucous membranes and skin turgor; monitor orthostatic blood pressure (lying, sitting, standing) every 4 h and more frequently if indicated (eg, vertigo); accompany to bathroom if self-induced vomiting suspected; review laboratory results and report abnormal values to primary clinician; educate about fluid intake needs, skin care, and positional changes to avoid orthostatic hypotension (15 mm Hg drop when upright, pulse increase of >15 beats/min); explore feelings and fears associated with increased fluid intake; promote oral hygiene |
| Fluid volume excess; risk for imbalanced fluid volume | Be aware of signs and symptom of fluid overload associated with refeeding (AN), monitor vital signs and weight regularly, note presence and degree of edema using standardized ratings (eg, 4-point scale) and patterns of urination, review laboratory data (blood urea nitrogen, creatinine, hemoglobin, hematocrit, electrolytes, urine specific gravity) and report abnormal findings to primary clinician, fluid restriction and/or monitoring if necessary (eg, patients who water load); assist patient to identify danger signs requiring notification of health care provider |
| Deficient knowledge regarding condition, prognosis, and/or treatment needs | Assess level of knowledge related to disorder, prognosis, nutritional, psychological, social and physiologic factors, treatment (eg, therapy, medications), and medical complications; assess readiness and ability to learn; identify support persons in need of information; use variety of teaching tools to engage patient (eg, didactic, audiovisual, printed materials); provide active role for patient in learning process; discuss laboratory findings, including purpose of test, normal values, and results; provide feedback and evaluation of learning; provide referral information, community resources, and additional informational resources before discharge (see **Table 5**) |
| Mood regulation, impaired | Assist patient to identify triggers for mood dysregulation, assess mood and associated psychological and physical symptoms, encourage patient to express feelings and listen empathically, identify coping mechanisms and provide education about options for improving emotion regulation and managing mood symptoms (eg, cognitive behavioral therapy, dialectical behavioral therapy), provide positive feedback and reinforcement, administer antidepressant or other medications as prescribed |

*(continued on next page)*

**Table 4**
*(continued)*

| Nursing Diagnoses | Potential Interventions (Determined by the Individual Case) |
|---|---|
| Noncompliance | Convey acceptance of patient separate from patient's behavior, discuss perception and understanding of disorder, listen to concerns and complaints, assess level of anxiety and sense of control, clarify value and belief system, assist to identify meaning and precipitants of resistant behavior; engage in mutual goal setting, identify treatment strategies more appealing and strategies likely to lead to noncompliance, contract for participation in care, provide information to patient, establish incremental goals |
| Nutrition, imbalanced: less than body requirements | Assess motivation for change; establish goal weight with treatment team and patient; establish daily caloric intake regimen for weight stabilization and eventual weight gain in collaboration with nutritionist; establish structure surrounding meals (eg, duration, setting, consequences if food not consumed), exercise patterns, weight measurements, and bathroom routines; assess understanding of nutritional needs; record fluid and food intake; calculate daily caloric intake; monitor vital signs including orthostatic blood pressure; review laboratory results and report abnormal finding to primary clinician; monitor meals; provide small quantities of food at more frequent intervals throughout the day (eg, with AN); administer nutritional supplements as indicated; provide small snacks at frequent intervals (eg, AN); in the event that a liquid diet via nasogastric tube is deemed necessary, carefully administer per orders and unit protocol; observe for 1 h after meals to deter purging; monitored use of bathroom if vomiting or excessive water intake is an actual or potential issue; explore feelings and emotions associated with food intake; refocus efforts directed at preoccupation with food; limit caffeine intake to 1 beverage daily; provide positive feedback for improved eating behavior; provide opportunities for feeling a sense of control (eg, offer choices), when possible; teach to recognize normal hunger and satiety signals |
| Obesity; overweight, risk for | Assess for motivation for change and knowledge of nutritional needs; ascertain perceptions of food and binge episodes; implement routine meal pattern; implement self-monitoring with food diaries to assist in identifying precipitating events, feelings, consequences, and other associated factors; calculate total caloric intake; assess degree of dietary restriction; provide positive reinforcement for successful nonbinge days; identify diversion activities to use in response to the urge to binge; identify high-risk situations for binge eating; identify normal hunger and satiety signals; assist in developing appropriate meal and exercise plan with care team; explore feelings and emotions associated with food intake |
| Pain, acute | Assess location, onset, duration, frequency, quality, precipitating and aggravating factors (use standardized self-report tool for pain); determine cause of pain (eg, gastritis, constipation); monitor vital signs; obtain history of previous experience with pain and methods of relief; encourage verbalization of pain; assist to identify pain prevention strategies (eg, abstinence of vomiting, relief of constipation) |

| | |
|---|---|
| Powerlessness | Determine perception of control; provide opportunities to express feelings and concerns; encourage questions; express hope for the patient; assist to identify strengths, assets, and past effective coping; identify areas beyond control and areas in which patient can actively participate; provide opportunity to make as many decisions as possible and as appropriate; minimize rules and reduce continuous observation as safety allows; model problem-solving techniques and explore new strategies; include patient in setting goals of care; allow to establish schedule of self-care activities; assist in setting incremental and achievable goals and provide positive reinforcement of successes |
| Self-esteem, situational low | Assist patient to identify contributing factors, encourage and provide positive reinforcement for independent decision-making and participation in treatment planning, encourage expression of feelings and emotions, provide reality testing to assist recognition of unrealistic self-perception, assist to identify strengths and positive self-attributes not related to body shape and weight, encourage positive references of self, redirect patient when comparing self to others, encourage socialization, refer to support group |
| Self-mutilation, risk for | Assess for impulsivity, unpredictability, and intense and uncontrolled anger; monitor patient closely and institute regular safety checks if indicated; assist to identify feelings and behaviors that precede urge to self-mutilate and consequences of self-mutilation (eg, perceived advantages and disadvantages); assist to express feelings appropriately; structure milieu to maintain open communication among staff and patients; remove dangerous objects from environment; assess for splitting or manipulation of staff or others; encourage involvement in plan of care; mobilize support systems; develop safety contract by which patient agrees to not self-mutilate in specified time frame (eg, next 8 h, with renewal if indicated before end of shift) |
| Suicide, risk for | Assign patient to a room close to the nursing station; do not leave patient alone if risk is high; spend time with the patient; assess potential for self-harm by asking directly about thoughts of killing self, plans, intent, and method; create and maintain safe environment (remove sharp items, glass, razor, scissors, ties, straps, belts); acknowledge reality of suicidal feelings; explain purpose and need for suicide precautions in a supportive manner; use contract that patient will not harm self during each shift and will remain in view of staff (renew contract before the start of next shift); monitor closely as energy increases and mood improves (greater risk to act on thoughts); encourage talking about feelings; closely monitor at times when staffing is anticipated to be low; help to identify hope; provide with as much control as possible within limits of providing safe environment; identify current and past strengths and successes; remain calm and state limits on inappropriate behavior; explore death fantasies when expressed; identify and engage support system; identify community resources; establish plan for seeking help in event of crisis |
| Trauma, risk for | Orient patient to environment, assure use of nonskid footwear, encourage adequate nutritional intake, implement exercise restrictions, administer calcium supplements as ordered, provide information and anticipatory guidance with regard to bone density testing procedures as ordered |

For additional resources see Ackley & Ladwig,[51] Herdman & Kamisturu,[52] and Townsend.[53]

been shown to predict short-term outcomes. Nasogastric feeding is used in life-threatening situations and is preferred to parenteral nutrition.[54,61] It is associated with significant risks for fluid overload and cardiac failure, and long-term use has not been shown to produce preferable outcomes.[54,62]

Establishment of structural and monitoring protocol is useful. Structure regarding meals and snacks is needed. Meals occur in a dining setting, if possible, and may require strict visual monitoring during and 1 hour after meals. For meals not eaten, missed calories are replaced with nutritional supplements. Time allotted for a meal is usually 30 minutes. Meal planning involves the patient in food selection.

Across treatment settings, weight assessment procedures vary in terms of time of day, frequency, and context.[63,64] Body weight measurements are obtained on admission after voiding and while in a hospital gown. Subsequent weights are obtained in an identical fashion. Patients with AN may revert to unusual measures to increase their weight (eg, excessive fluid intake) before weighing.[63] Weights are reassessed immediately when unexpected changes occur. Few empirical data exist on whether or not to inform the patient his or her weight, although both approaches seem to be used.[65]

### Exercise

For patients with AN, exercise is restricted on admission because it defeats the goal of weight gain. Eventually, supervised exercise is gradually reintroduced directed at health promotion, fitness, and prevention of bone loss rather than weight loss.[54]

### Medications

Medications may be indicated in the presence of significant comorbidity. To date there is no medication approved by the US Food and Drug Administration (FDA) for the treatment of AN. Low-weight states may make these patients more vulnerable to side effects. In preliminary studies, olanzapine has been associated with weight gain in AN.[66] To date, fluoxetine is the only FDA-approved drug to treat BN. Antidepressant agents have been shown to decrease frequency of binges,[67] with selective serotonin reuptake inhibitors usually having the more favorable side-effect profile. Bupropion hydrochloride and bupropion hydrobromide are specifically contraindicated in persons with current or history of AN or BN given observations of associated seizures.[68] Lisdexamfetamine dimesylate was recently approved by the FDA for the treatment of BED.

### Milieu

The inpatient environment is often highly structured to encourage behavior modification and cognitive restructuring. Family involvement is encouraged, particularly for younger patients,[69] including participation in family therapy sessions and meals. Sometimes restrictions are needed to prevent compensatory behaviors or binges. Clear communication between staff is essential.

### Discharge Planning

Discharge planning, begins on admission and is essential for providing the patient, family, and subsequent treatment team information about aftercare plans.[56] Plans regarding level of care, treatments, medications, and the names, contact information, and appointments for aftercare providers need to be conveyed. Residential care or outpatient individual therapy is often recommended. Group therapy, family therapy, and nutritional counseling are useful therapies to consider. Additionally, plans for medical monitoring of physical health and/or medication response are a consideration. With consent of the patient, a discharge summary is made available to aftercare providers to facilitate continuity of care.[56] Additional resources are listed in **Table 5**.

| Table 5 Potential resource[a] (representative listing) | |
| --- | --- |
| Organization | Web Site |
| Academy for Eating Disorders | http://www.aedweb.org |
| Alliance for Eating Disorder Awareness | http://www.allianceforeatingdisorders.com |
| Andrea's Voice | http://andreasvoice.org |
| Binge Eating Disorder Association | http://bedaonline.com |
| British Columbia Eating Disorders Association | http://webhome.idirect.com/~bceda/index.html |
| Compulsive Eaters Anonymous- HOW | http://www.ceahow.org |
| Eating Disorders Anonymous | http://www.eatingdisordersanonymous.org |
| Eating Disorders Coalition | http://www.eatingdisorderscoalition.org |
| Eating Disorders Referral Information Center | http://www.edreferral.com |
| Food Addicts Anonymous | http://www.foodaddictsanonymous.org |
| Healthy Choices for Mind and Body | http://www.healthychoicesformindandbody.org |
| International Association of Eating Disorders Professionals | http://www.iaedp.com |
| Maudsley Parents | http://www.maudsleyparents.org |
| Multiservice Eating Disorders Association | http://www.medainc.org |
| National Association to Advance Fat Acceptance | http://www.naafa.org |
| National Association of Anorexia Nervosa and Associated Disorders | http://www.anad.org |
| National Eating Disorders Association | http://www.nationaleatingdisorders.org |
| National Eating Disorder Information Centre | http://www.nedic.ca |
| National Institute of Mental Health | http://www.nimh.nih.gov |
| Overeaters Anonymous | http://www.overeatersanonymous.org |

[a] Content of Web sites can be variable and should be assessed for accuracy and appropriateness.[70]

## SUMMARY

Effective nursing care for hospitalized patients with an eating disorder is based on a comprehensive assessment. Hospitalization is appropriate for most acute patients experiencing impaired functioning, severe malnutrition or comorbidity, or who are at increased risk for medical instability. Inpatient nursing care is tailored to the individual's needs to optimize health status.

## REFERENCES

1. Hudson JI, Hiripi E, Pope HG, et al. The prevalence and correlates of eating disorders in the National Comorbidity Survey Replication. Biol Psychiatry 2007;61: 348–58.

2. Arcelus J, Mitchell AJ, Wales J, et al. Mortality rates in patients with anorexia nervosa and other eating disorders: a meta-analysis of 36 studies. Arch Gen Psychiatry 2011;68:724–31.

3. Smink FRE, van Hoeken D, Hoek HW. Epidemiology of eating disorders: Incidence, prevalence and mortality rates. Curr Psychiatry Rep 2012;14:406–14.

4. Kessler RC, Berglund PA, Chiu WT, et al. The prevalence and correlates of binge eating disorder in the World Health Organization World Mental Health Surveys. Biol Psychiatry 2013;73:904–14.

5. Jennings KM, Kelly-Weeder S, Wolfe BE. Binge eating among racial minority groups in the United States: an integrative review. J Am Psychiatr Nurses Assoc 2015;21:117–25.

6. Culbert KM, Racine SE, Klump KL. Research review: what we have learned about the causes of eating disorders – a synthesis of sociocultural, psychological, and biological research. J Child Psychol Psychiatry 2015;56:1141–64.

7. Lobera IJ, Rios PB, Casals OG. Parenting styles and eating disorders. J Psychiatr Ment Health Nurs 2011;18:728–35.

8. Ciccolo EBF. Exploring experience of family relations by patients with anorexia nervosa and bulimia nervosa using a projective family test. Psychol Rep 2008; 103:231–42.

9. Amianto F, Ercole R, Marzola E, et al. Parents' personality clusters and eating disordered daughters' personality and psychopathy. Psychiatry Res 2015; 230(1):19–27.

10. American Psychiatric Association. Diagnostic and statistical manual of mental disorders. 5th edition. Arlington (VA): American Psychiatric Association; 2013.

11. Ulfvebrand S, Birgegard A, Norring C, et al. Psychiatric comorbidity in women and men with eating disorders results from a large clinical database. Psychiatry Res 2015;230:294–9.

12. Muehlenkamp JJ, Claes L, Smits D, et al. Nonsuicidal self-injury in eating disordered patients: a test of a conceptual model. Psychiatry Res 2011;188:102–8.

13. Zalar B, Weber U, Sernec K. Aggression and impulsivity with impulsive behaviours in patients with purgative anorexia and bulimia nervosa. Psychiatr Danub 2011;23(1):27–33.

14. Caslini M, Bartoli F, Crocamo C, et al. Disentangling the association between child abuse and eating disorders: a systematic review and meta-analysis. Psychosom Med 2016;78(1):79–90.

15. Reas DL, Ro O, Karterud S, et al. Eating disorders in a large clinical sample of men and women with personality disorders. Int J Eat Disord 2013;46:801–9.

16. Becker DF, Grilo CM. Comorbidity of mood and substance use disorders in patients with binge-eating disorder: associations with personality disorder and eating disorder pathology. J Psychosom Res 2015;79:159–64.

17. Twomey CD, Baldwin DS, Hopfe M, et al. A systematic review of the predictors of health service utilization by adults with mental disorders in the UK. BMJ Open 2015;5:e007575.

18. Kermarrec S, Kabuth B, Rat A-C, et al. The outcome of adolescent-onset anorexia nervosa: a study of 144 cases. Health 2014;6:1883–93.

19. Steinhausen H-C. The outcome of anorexia nervosa in the 20th century. Am J Psychiatry 2002;159:1284–93.

20. Carter JC, Mercer-Lynn KB, Norwood SJ, et al. A prospective study of predictors of relapse in anorexia nervosa: implications for relapse prevention. Psychiatry Res 2012;200:518–23.

21. Grilo CM, Pagano ME, Skodol AE, et al. Natural course of bulimia nervosa and of eating disorder not otherwise specified: 5-year prospective study of remission, relapses, and the effects of personality disorder psychopathology. J Clin Psychiatry 2007;68:738–46.

22. Keel PK, Gravener JA, Joiner TE, et al. Twenty-year follow-up of bulimia nervosa and related eating disorders not otherwise specified. Int J Eat Disord 2010;43: 492–7.
23. Steinhausen H-C, Weber S. The outcome of bulimia nervosa: findings from one-quarter century of research. Am J Psychiatry 2009;166:1331–41.
24. Olmsted MP, MacDonald DE, McFarlane T, et al. Predictors of rapid relapse in bulimia nervosa. Int J Eat Disord 2015;48:337–40.
25. Wonderlich SA, Gordon KH, Mitchell JE, et al. The validity and utility of binge eating disorder. Int J Eat Disord 2009;42:687–705.
26. Zugai JS, Stein-Parbury J, Roche M. Therapeutic alliance in mental health nursing: an evolutionary concept analysis. Issues Ment Health Nurs 2015;36: 249–57.
27. Zaitsoff S, Pullmer R, Cyr M, et al. The role of the therapeutic alliance in eating disorder treatment outcomes: A systematic review. Eat Disord 2015;23:99–114.
28. King SJ, Turner de S. Caring for adolescent females with anorexia nervosa: registered nurses' perspective. J Adv Nurs 2000;32:139–47.
29. Snell L, Crowe M, Jordan J. Maintaining a therapeutic connection: nursing in an inpatient eating disorder unit. J Clin Nurs 2010;19:351–8.
30. Abbate-Daga G, Amianto F, Delsedime N, et al. Resistance to treatment in eating disorders: a critical challenge. BMC Psychiatry 2013;13:292.
31. Bates CF. "I am a waste of breath, of space, of time": metaphors of self in a pro-anorexia group. Qual Health Res 2015;25:189–204.
32. Vall E, Wade TD. Predictors of treatment outcome in individuals with eating disorders: a systematic review and meta-analysis. Int J Eat Disord 2015;48:946–71.
33. Menatti AR, DeBoer LBH, Weeks JW, et al. Social anxiety and associations with eating psychopathology: mediating effects of fears of evaluation. Body Image 2015;14:20–8.
34. Leonidas C, Santos MA. Family relations in eating disorders: the genogram as instrument of assessment. Cien Saude Colet 2015;20:1435–47.
35. Carney CP, Andersen AE. Eating disorders: guide to medical evaluation and complications. Psychiatr Clin North Am 1996;19:657–79.
36. Westmoreland P, Krantz MJ, Mehler PS. Medical complications of anorexia nervosa and bulimia. Am J Med 2016;129(1):30–7.
37. Sato Y, Fukudo S. Gastrointestinal symptoms and disorders in patients with eating disorders. Clin J Gastroenterol 2015;8:255–63.
38. Fernstrom MH, Weltzin TE, Neuberger S, et al. Twenty-four-hour food intake in patients with anorexia nervosa and in health control subjects. Biol Psychiatry 1994; 36:696–702.
39. U.S. Department of Agriculture and Department of Health and Human Services. Dietary guidelines for Americans 2010. 7th edition. Washington, DC: U.S. Government Printing Office; 2010.
40. Elran-Barak R, Sztainer M, Goldschmidt AB, et al. Dietary restriction behaviors and binge eating in anorexia nervosa, bulimia nervosa, and binge eating disorder: trans-diagnostic examination of the restraint model. Eat Behav 2015;18: 192–6.
41. Wolfe BE, Baker CW, Smith AT, et al. Validity and utility of the current definition of binge eating. Int J Eat Disord 2009;42:674–86.
42. U.S. Department of Health and Human Services. 2008 physical activity guidelines for Americans. Washington, DC: U.S. Government Printing Office; 2008.
43. Kelly AC, Vimalakanthan K, Carter JC. Understanding the roles of self-esteem, self-compassion, and fear of self-compassion in eating disorder pathology: an

examination of female students and eating disorder patients. Eat Behav 2014;15: 388–91.

44. Pearl RL, White MA, Grilo CM. Overvaluation of shape and weight as a mediator between self-esteem and weight bias internalization among patients with binge eating disorder. Eat Behav 2014;15:259–61.

45. Cash TF, Deagle EA. The nature and extent of body-image disturbances in anorexia nervosa and bulimia nervosa: a meta-analysis. Int J Eat Disord 1997; 22:107–25.

46. Lewer M, Nasrawi N, Schroeder D, et al. Body image disturbance in binge eating disorder: a comparison of obese patients with and without binge eating disorder regarding cognitive, behavioral and perceptual component of body image. Eat Weight Disord 2015. [Epub ahead of print].

47. Duarte C, Pinto-Gouveia J, Ferreira C. Escaping from body image shame and harsh self-criticism: exploration of underlying mechanisms of binge eating. Eat Behav 2014;15:638–43.

48. Goldschmidt AB, Hilbert A, Manwaring JL, et al. The significance of shape and weight in binge eating disorder. Behav Res Ther 2010;48:187–93.

49. Kuczmarski RJ, Ogden CL, Guo SS, et al. 2000 CDC growth charts for the United States: methods and development. National Center for Health Statistics. Vital Health Stat 11 2002;(246):1–190.

50. Pinheiro AP, Thornton LM, Plotonicov KH, et al. Patterns of menstrual disturbance in eating disorders. Int J Eat Disord 2007;40:424–34.

51. Ackley BJ, Ladwig GB. Nursing diagnosis handbook: an evidence-based guide to planning care. 10th edition. Maryland Height (MO): Mosby, Elsevier Inc; 2014.

52. Herdman TH, Kamitsuru S, editors. NANDA international nursing diagnoses: definitions & classification, 2015-2017. Oxford (United Kingdom): Wiley Blackwell; 2014.

53. Townsend MC. Psychiatric nursing: assessment, care plans, and medications. 9th edition. Philadelphia: FA Davis; 2014.

54. American Psychiatric Association. Practice guidelines for the treatment of patients with eating disorders. 3rd edition. Washington, DC: American Psychiatric Association; 2006.

55. Society for Adolescent Health and Medicine. Position paper of the Society for Adolescent Health and Medicine: medical management of restrictive eating disorders in adolescents and young adults. J Adolesc Health 2015;56:121–5.

56. Academy for Eating Disorders. Clinical practice recommendations for residential and inpatient eating disorder programs. Deerfield (IL): Academy for Eating Disorders; 2012.

57. Golden NH, Jacobson MS, Sterling WM, et al. Treatment goal weight in adolescents with anorexia nervosa: use of BMI percentiles. Int J Eat Disord 2008;41: 301–6.

58. Khan LUR, Ahmed J, Khan S, et al. Refeeding syndrome: a literature review. Gastroenterol Res Pract 2011;2011. Available at: http://www.hindawi.com/journals/grp/2011/410971. Accessed November 24, 2015.

59. Lund BC, Hernandez ER, Yates WR, et al. Rate of inpatient weight restoration predicts outcome in anorexia nervosa. Int J Eat Disord 2009;42:301–5.

60. Kaplan AS, Walsh BT, Olmsted M, et al. The slippery slope: prediction of successful weight maintenance in anorexia nervosa. Psychol Med 2009;39:1037–45.

61. Rosen DS. The Committee on Adolescence. Identification and management of eating disorders in children and adolescents. Pediatrics 2010;126:1240–5.

62. Golden NH, Katzman DK, Kreipe RE, et al. Eating disorders in adolescents: position paper of the Society for Adolescent Medicine. J Adolesc Health 2003;33: 496–503.

63. Jaffa T, Davies S, Sardesai A. What patients with anorexia nervosa should wear when they are being weighed: Report of two pilot studies. Eur Eat Disord Rev 2011;19:368–70.

64. Schwartz BI, Mansbach JM, Marion JG, et al. Variations in admission practices for adolescents with anorexia nervosa: a North American sample. J Adolesc Health 2008;43:425–31.

65. Forbush KT, Richardson JH, Bohrer BK. Clinicians' practices regarding blinding versus open weighing among patients with eating disorders. Int J Eat Disord 2015;48:905–11.

66. McElroy SL, Guerdjikova AI, Mori N, et al. Psychopharmacologic treatment of eating disorders: emerging findings. Curr Psychiatry Rep 2015;17(5):35.

67. Flament MF, Bissada H, Spettigue W. Evidence-based pharmacotherapy of eating disorders. Int J Neuropsychopharmacol 2011;15:189–207.

68. Bupropion. Available at: http://www.pdr.net. Accessed November 30, 2015.

69. Le Grange D, Lock J, Loeb K, et al. Academy for eating disorders position paper: the role of the family in eating disorders. Int J Eat Disord 2009;43:1–5.

70. Smith AT, Kelly-Weeder S, Engel J, et al. Quality of eating disorders websites: what adolescents and their families need to know. J Child Adolesc Psychiatr Nurs 2011;24:33–7.

# Dual Diagnosis
## Coexisting Substance Use Disorders and Psychiatric Disorders

Deborah Antai-Otong, MS, APRN, PMHCNS-BC, FAAN[a],
Kristine Theis, FNP, MSN, RN[b], Dee Dee Patrick, MS, RN, CARN[c],*

### KEYWORDS

- Dual diagnosis • Co-occurring • Addiction
- Screening Brief Intervention Referral and Treatment (SBIRT) • Cravings
- Motivational interviewing

### KEY POINTS

- Coexisting substance use disorders (SUDs) and psychiatric disorders are mutually injurious and complicate treatment outcomes and prognosis.
- Gender issues must be addressed when screening for SUDs and psychiatric disorders.
- Screening Brief Interventions and Referral to Treatment is an evidence-based approach that helps to identify, mitigate, and reduce risky substance use behaviors.
- Psychopharmacologic and psychotherapeutic approaches have proven efficacy in the treatment of dual diagnoses.

### INTRODUCTION

A dual diagnosis is characterized by a substance use disorder (SUD) and psychiatric disorder that occur simultaneously. These disorders affect the lives of individuals and their families across the life span regardless of age, gender, race, ethnicity, socioeconomic status, culture, and spiritual beliefs. The high incidence of people with a dual diagnosis is well documented. According to the findings from the National Survey on Drug Use and Health[1] about 45% of individuals with an SUD have a coexisting psychiatric disorder, and of the 17.5 million Americans, 8% of adults have experienced a serious psychiatric disorder in the past year. Of these, an estimated 4 million people also dealt with a co-occurring SUDs.

---

This article is an update of an article previously published in Nursing Clinics of North America, Volume 38, Issue 1, March 2003.

Disclosures: None.

[a] Department of Veterans Affairs, Veterans Integrated Service Networks-(VISN-17), 2301 E. Lamar Boulevard, Arlington, TX 76006, USA; [b] Boise VAMC, Boise, ID, USA; [c] 21363 Settlers Pond Drive, Frankfort, IL 60423-7978, USA

* Corresponding author.

*E-mail address:* Dmp0513@aol.com

Coexisting SUD and psychiatric disorders are mutually injurious and complicate treatment outcomes and prognosis, increase hospitalizations, delay symptom remission, and heighten the risk of suicide attempts.[2,3] These disorders are also the principal causes of related morbidity (ie, medical complications related to chronic substance use) and mortality among women and the second highest among men.[4] Negative treatment outcomes are also associated with the large number of patients with a dual diagnosis who do not receive treatment of both disorders. Approximately 34% of this population receive psychiatric care, 2% receive treatment of SUDs, and 12% receive care for a dual diagnosis.[1] Adverse treatment outcomes are also linked to inadequate clinician training and awareness about integrated screening and evaluation to rule out separate disorders. At present, there is a paucity of treatment research that guides the management of dual diagnosis. The stigma of seeking services for SUD and psychiatric disorders continues to impede access to needed services and heightens the risk of ineffective coping behaviors, such as self-medication. Self-medication used to manage psychiatric disorders presents a substantial risk of SUD. Self-medication serves to assuage intense emotional distress.[5,6] There are growing concerns about the number of patients who seek help in primary care and mental health settings with coexisting SUDs and psychiatric disorders.

## PREVALENCE

Data from the National Survey on Drug Use and Health[1] reveals that most people with a dual diagnosis are gainfully employed and that men are 2 times more likely than women to have a dual diagnosis. However, women were more likely to have had a serious psychiatric disorder in the past 12 months. Historically, alcohol was the primary drug of choice for half of the people with a dual diagnosis. However, during the 2000s the largest increase for a single substance has been non–medical use prescription opiates, such as oxycodone. Of this population, approximately 21% of patients were addicted to prescription opiates, which is an increase of 13% in the past decade.[1] More recent data confirm the high use of nonmedical prescription opiates, particularly among women.[7] Conclusions from this survey and other data suggest that the increase in nonmedical prescription opiate use is a significant contributor to dual diagnosis in patients with coexisting psychiatric and physical disorders.[8] The recent upsurge in the use of nonmedical use opiates remains a clinical challenge to nurses and other providers caring for patients with coexisting psychiatric and physical disorders.

More recent data from epidemiologic surveys on alcohol abuse and related disorders[3] further support the prevalence of these disorders and concluded that alcohol abuse disorder, posttraumatic disorders, and unipolar depression were the most common coexisting psychiatric disorders, particularly among vulnerable populations. Vulnerable populations associated with these disorders include family history of SUD, younger age, female gender, combat exposure, and a history of childhood abuse.[3,9]

This article provides an overview of salient clinical issues involving coexisting SUDs and psychiatric disorders (dual diagnosis). It highlights the role of psychiatric mental health and addiction nurses in the treatment of these complex disorders, which includes early identification, integrated screening, and assessment of patients who present with a dual diagnosis. It describes the powerful properties of cocaine and other drugs and the role of cue-related memories in sustaining addiction and complicating the treatment of these disorders. Dual diagnosis treatment that integrates pharmacologic and psychotherapeutic approaches is also reviewed.

## INTEGRATED SCREENING AND ASSESSMENT OF SUBSTANCE USE DISORDER AND PSYCHIATRIC DISORDERS
### Integrated Screening and Assessment

Despite barriers to treatment there is growing evidence that these patients may benefit from integrated treatment modalities that target and treat both of these distinct disorders.[10,11] Determining the appropriate dual diagnosis care is a complex process that generally begins with screening and medical stabilization to assess the course of care and interventions. Active SUD interferes with effective management of psychiatric disorders primarily because of the difficulty in distinguishing symptoms, such as psychosis and anxiety, that are drug induced from the primary symptoms of psychiatric and disorders. Conventional treatment of a dual diagnosis begins with an integrated screening and evaluation process that occurs within a context in which both disorders are assessed. The following discussion focuses on screening and brief interventions. Establishing rapport and conveying empathy and concern enable nurses to engage these patients in a therapeutic relationship. Some patients feel embarrassed or ashamed of their drug use history. A nonjudgmental and accepting approach creates an environment that puts the patients at ease and makes them more comfortable when answering questions concerning their substance use, legal history involving illicit drug use, and psychiatric history. Patient engagement is a key feature of therapeutic relationships because it supports self-directed partnerships and facilitates confidence in the patients' decisions to seek treatment.

An often overlooked clinical issue that contributes to the complexity and treatment of dual diagnoses is a failure to screen for SUD while screening for psychiatric disorders. Because of the high morbidity and mortality associated with these disorders it is vital for nurses to screen all patients for dual diagnosis. Screening all patients helps nurses identify high-risk groups and vulnerable populations. The US Preventive Services Task Force has made recommendation for alcohol and illicit drug screening and behavioral interventions for more than 2 decades.[12] Although screening and brief interventions are commonly conducted in primary care settings, the focus is primarily on risk or harmful drinking and singular interventions. *This focus is* generally ineffective in treatments for alcohol use disorders.

Regardless, screening can occur in any health care setting and can have a meaningful effect on motivating patients to consider treatment. The Screening and Brief Intervention and Referral to Treatment (SBIRT) is a voluntary process that requires patients to be active participants.[13] Implementation of this practice has been used extensively in primary settings to identify patients with an SUD. SBIRT is an evidence-based approach used to identify, mitigate, and prevent risky substance use behaviors. Screening tools, such as the cutting down, annoyed, guilty, eye opener (CAGE) questionnaire and the Alcohol Use Disorders Identification Test (AUDIT-C)[13–16] can be used to assess alcohol use and risky drinking patterns. Brief behavioral interventions involve short dialogue and feedback with the patients about adverse consequences of risky behaviors and harm reduction, based on answers concerning the impact of the SUD on the patient's life. In the case of women who are pregnant or may become pregnant, brief intervention needs to include a discussion about the harmful effects of SUDs on the unborn child, and infant if they are breastfeeding.

Motivational interviewing skills put the onus on the patient for making changes and use empathy to bolster self-confidence and commitment to reduce the risk of substance use behaviors.[17] Following the screening and brief intervention process the patients may need a more extensive biopsychosocial evaluation and treatment. Screening results and treatment options must be discussed with the patients.[13,14] If the patient has active symptoms of a dual diagnosis (eg, intoxication, psychosis) and the nurse has difficulty distinguishing distinct symptoms of each disorder, the nurse needs to consult with appropriate providers and refer the patient for a comprehensive psychiatric and medical evaluation and medical stabilization.

## Making a Diagnosis

Medical clearance involves a complete history and physical; a battery of laboratory studies, including renal, hepatic, hematologic (ie, complete blood count, mean corpuscle volume), urinalysis, urine drug screen testing for coexisting SUDs, and endocrine studies (eg, thyroid function tests). Signs of drug toxicity warrant a baseline electrocardiogram. Management of acute medical conditions is a priority and should be tailored to address the severity of the patient's presenting symptoms. Additional assessment data required to complete the diagnosis come from the comprehensive biopsychosocial assessment.

Major components of the biopsychosocial assessment include a mental status examination, reasons for seeking treatment at this time, past history of treatment of both disorders, and current medications (including prescription, over-the-counter, and herbal and dietary supplements with psychoactive properties). In circumstances in which the nurse doubts the patient's response to questions concerning drug use or psychiatric treatment, it is essential to ask approval to request information from close family members or providers. Additional areas that need to be assessed include:

- Present and past history of cravings (eg, ask whether patients remember a time when they had such strong urges to use the drug that they were unable to focus on other things). A positive response is thought to predict relapse and may dissuade the patient from trying to quit.
- Adherence to treatment regimen, including medications for a psychiatric or medical disorder.
- Current social support, including current relationships and employment history.
- Legal history, including relationship to substance use.
- History of menstrual cycle, pregnancies, age of menopause, and contraception use (history of mood changes during menstrual cycles and menopause).
- Current and past history of substance use patterns, including last time used, previous treatment of SUDs, and psychiatric disorders.
- Improved quality of life.
- Present safety level.
- Current and past history of suicidal/homicidal ideations, current or past thoughts, intent, means, and prior history and treatment.
- Trauma history; also determine whether there is a relationship with substance use (ie, self-medication).

As previously discussed, initial treatment planning involves stabilization of the SUD followed by treating the psychiatric disorder to reduce exacerbation and relapse. Before initiating treatment, a possible dual diagnosis must be confirmed based on Diagnostic and Statistical Manual of Mental Disorders, Fifth Edition (DSM-V) criteria for an SUDs and psychiatric disorder.[18] In 2013, the American Psychiatric Association[18] redefined diagnostic criteria for substance use by categorizing SUDs in a single continuum. The new chapter is entitled "Substance-related and Addictive Disorders". Criteria of tolerance and withdrawal were eliminated, and craving and abuse symptoms, plus a new graded severity classification, were added. A core characteristic of an SUDs is a cluster of cognitive, behavioral, and physiologic symptoms showing continued use of the substance despite significant substance-related problems.

SUDs are categorized as mild, moderate, or severe, which is determined by the number of diagnostic criteria. A specific SUD parallels the drug properties, risky use, and level of global impairment and morbidity.[18] Criteria for psychiatric disorders are associated with specific symptoms associated with these disorders (eg, major depression, bipolar disorder, schizophrenia). Specific symptoms are found in each chapter listed with a DSM-V diagnosis. When a dual diagnosis is confirmed and the patient expresses motivation and willingness to change and participate in treatment the nurses need to refer the patient to appropriate providers for further evaluation and treatment. Motivation for change occurs over a continuum of readiness in which the clients progress through the various stages of changes. The goal of care must be to treat the patients for both disorders in tandem using a person-centered approach.

## TREATMENT CONSIDERATIONS
### Dual Diagnosis Treatment Modalities

Emerging changes in the treatment of coexisting SUDs and psychiatric disorders have occurred the past 10 to 15 years. Research continues to link complex biological, neuroanatomic and neuroendocrine, gender, and genetic biomarkers to dual diagnoses. During this period there has also been a surge in the incidence of SUDs in women that has led to a greater emphasis on the impact of gender in the symptoms and treatment of these disorders. Notably, researchers have discovered that women experience unique responses to drugs that are associated with hormonal factors, such as menstrual cycles, menopause, pregnancy, and breastfeeding.[7,18] Frequently, women report that their reasons for using drugs include self-medication to cope with the stress of childrearing and work responsibilities and caring for aging parents. In addition, they complain of concerns about their personal appearance and the need to take drugs for weight control, fatigue, and chronic pain problems[18] **Box 1** lists gender-related issues associated with SUDs. Regardless of the reasons why women use drugs to self-medicate and manage stressful situations or deal with depression and anxiety, similar to outcomes involving men, continual use of drugs heightens the

---

**Box 1**
**Gender-related issues associated with SUDs**

*Women:*

- May have more drug cravings and be more likely to relapse after discharge from treatment
- Hormonal mood changes may contribute to risk of relapse
- May develop adverse psychiatric and physical consequence sooner than men despite consuming less amounts of drugs
- Hormonal changes may affect the metabolism of some drugs and medications
- More likely to experience trauma than men
- Relationship problems, death of a significant other, and other losses may contribute to a dual diagnosis
- More likely to experience mood and anxiety disorders when using certain drugs
- More likely to abuse pain medications

"Every 3 minutes, a woman goes to the emergency room for prescription painkiller misuse or abuse."[7]

risk of adverse consequences (eg, suicide risk). These underpinnings have a significant impact on cognitive and behavioral responses to cravings and drug-seeking behaviors despite adverse consequences.[19]

Addiction is considered a progressive and compulsive brain disorder, and is characterized by recurrent cravings and relapse and cue-induced drug-seeking behaviors that frequently occur despite prolonged periods of abstinence.[20] Cravings are partially caused by the powerful internal memories or exposure to triggers (external stimuli) associated with the substance, drug-seeking behaviors, and drug-using behaviors. In addition, they are linked to high morbidity and mortality. Cravings are principal features of addiction and they are implicated in symptom maintenance of SUD and relapse, and are a biomarker for treatment. Scientists submit that effective treatment of SUDs are approaches that mitigate or interrupt the intensity of cues associated with memory consolidation (sustained memory storage).[19] Reducing the strength of these cue-drug memories may also decrease the number of factors that induce cravings and relapse and aid in the treatment of addiction.

Treatment goals need to be person centered and tailored to the patient's readiness and stage of change, and must ensure that the patients have the education and encouragement to make personal decisions about their care[4] (**Box 2**). During the course of treatment and follow-up, patients should be closely evaluated and monitored because of the potential impact of SUDs on coexisting psychiatric disorders and interactions with the medications used to treat them.[21,22] Depending on the SUD and psychiatric disorder, patients need to be educated about pharmacologic and/or psychotherapeutic treatment options so they can make personal decisions and actively participate in their care.[4] It is paramount that treatment reflects the patient's strengths, abilities, preferences, and motivation for change. The process of change requires that patients accept treatment and begin a recovery-based program for dual diagnosis.

---

**Box 2**
**Stages of change**

Precontemplation: the patient is not interested in change and lacks insight and awareness of the need to change.

Contemplation: the patient recognizes the negative and positive aspects of substance use, but is ambivalent about change and at this point unwilling to make a commitment to change. The patient is amenable to reading educational materials about negative consequences of continued substance use.

Preparation: at this stage the patient is ready to change and begin the journey of recovery. The patient takes steps to call for an appointment to address substance use.

Action: the patient attempts new behaviors, but these are not well established. This stage involves the first effective steps to change.

Maintenance: the patient develops and uses new coping and *problem-solving* behaviors on a long- term basis.

Relapse: reverting to previous maladaptive behaviors.

*Data from* Prochaska JO, DiClemente CC. The transtheoretical approach: crossing traditional boundaries of therapy. Homewood (IL): Dow Jones Irwin; 1984; and Department of Health and Human Services, Substance Abuse and Mental Health Services Administration. Brief interventions and therapies for substance abuse KAP Keys for clinicians based on TIP 34. HHS publication no. (SMA) 153601. 2015. Available at: http://store.samhsa.gov/product/Brief-Interventions-and-Therapies-for-Substance-Abuse/BackInStock/SMA15-3601. Accessed December 3, 2015.

## Pharmacologic Interventions

Biomarkers for treatment include pharmacologic and psychotherapeutic approaches that facilitate the development of adaptive coping skills to manage stress and triggers associated with cue-drug–related memories.[19] Compelling evidence suggests that drugs that strengthen the medial prefrontal cortex control over cravings and drug-seeking behaviors are implicated in the treatment of SUDs and addictive disorders. This brain region is primarily involved in executive functioning and is implicated in planning complex behavior: decision making, goal directing, and tempering social behavior.[23] The specific medications prescribed are determined by each disorder and the patient's preference.

A preponderance of research points to the success of antidepressants used in the treatment of coexisting depressive disorders and SUD, and reveals modest results that were associated with side effects and increased risk of toxicity. Other studies indicate that naltrexone and selective serotonin reuptake inhibitors have proven usefulness in the treatment of patients with a depressive disorder and alcohol use.[24] Atypical antipsychotics, such as quetiapine and clozapine, have proven efficacy in the treatment of schizophrenia and SUD, such as those involving alcohol, cocaine, and amphetamines. In the case of opioid use and psychiatric disorders, medications that mitigate cravings and drug-seeking behaviors are showing promising results. $N$-methyl-D-aspartate antagonists[25] and protein synthesis inhibitors are examples of these agents.[26] Purportedly, the efficacy of these drugs derives from their ability to reduce the intensity of cue-drug–related drug-seeking and drug-consumption behavior. These findings also emphasize the importance of integrated treatment that combines pharmacologic and psychotherapeutic interventions, such motivational interviewing.

## Psychotherapeutic Interventions

Motivational interviewing has been shown to be effective in working with patients with a dual diagnosis. Its emphasis on placing the responsibility for change directly on the patient works hand in hand with individualized models for change. Within this framework there is reduced focus on confrontation, which is more acceptable with this particular population. Resistance on the part of the patient is viewed as an interpersonal behavior pattern that is influenced by the nurse psychotherapist's behavior. The personal concerns of the patient are elicited, providing the nurse psychotherapist with leverage to challenge denial. Reflection is used to amplify the patient's discrepancies and enhance motivation for change, and for patients to take an active part and responsibility in their own treatment progress.[17]

Patients with a dual diagnosis who perceive change as a threatening and negative experience may be reluctant and uncomfortable with psychiatric nurses and other providers who suggest strategies for changes. If the desired outcomes of these changes seem unlikely or possible only in the distant future, commitment will not be sustained. Patients with SUDs, by the nature of their disorders, respond to and expect immediate gratification activated by cue-drug memories. Strategies for behavioral change need to include a supportive relationship and should begin by targeting achievable, short-term goals that build confidence. In the case of depression, PTSD, and anxiety disorders, cognitive-behavior therapies have proven efficacy.[27] An accepting approach that focuses on the patient's strengths, wishes, and preferences, and that uses empathy rather than authority, are critical to patients with a dual diagnosis.

Problem-solving processes are elicited from the patients and significant others. The perceptions of the patient seeking treatment are explored without making any attempts to correct them. Placing attention and the onus for change on the patient is instrumental in achieving and sustaining significant change. Helpful psychoeducation topics available to the patient include defining specific psychiatric disorders and SUDs in patient-friendly terms, discussing triggers for relapse, identifying good and bad drugs, contingency management, and discussing family issues and concerns. Benefits of family-based interventions in the treatment of a dual diagnosis include strengthening relationships, being able to express their feelings and thoughts in a safe environment, and learning how to support patients during stressful times while reinforcing adaptive coping behaviors.[28]

It is widely acknowledged that an increase in perceived stress is one of the most frequent causes of exacerbation of symptoms of SUDs and psychiatric disorders. The importance of didactic training in ways to deal with stress cannot be overemphasized. Teaching behavioral techniques as simple as deep breathing exercises to deal with an increase in anxiety is not only practical but also effective. The significance of stress management and other relaxation techniques cannot be overemphasized.

Patients with dual diagnosis often lack the quality adaptive coping and problem-solving skills necessary to effectively mitigate stress and exacerbation of symptoms associated with each disorder. Teaching social skills and behavioral strategies for limiting stressful interactions and providing information regarding how to establish and maintain healthy interpersonal skills, and to effectively handle activities of daily living, are important psychoeducational modules. Attendees are encouraged to ask questions, share personal experiences, and express ideas on ways to cope with problems that impede their recovery. Patients with a history of relapsing are especially vulnerable to stressful situations and should take steps to anticipate stressful and high-risk situations, manage triggers, and develop stress management skills that help them handle unexpected stressful encounters and avoid reverting to previous ineffective coping behaviors.[13,29]

Teaching behavioral techniques as simple as deep breathing exercise to deal with increased anxiety is not only practical but also effective. A 30-minute psychoeducation group allows ample time to educate patients about the importance of taking medications as prescribed and discuss the side effects to report. These gatherings also provide opportunities to discuss personal reactions or fears about medications, build trust, and gain support from peers. Role playing or getting an audience involved in discussions about how they would react if they saw others drinking or engaging in risky behaviors is paramount to the development of sound coping skills. Patients with a dual diagnosis need to be able to apply what they learn to real-life situations. These interactions enable patients to relate to each other better than didactic lectures given *their shared experiences* about the harms of substance use or non-adherence to medication for psychiatric disorders.

Using written materials with groups and individual contacts has been found to be more effective than verbal instructions alone. It is also imperative to assess the learning styles and preferences of each patient to determine the best approach to educate them about health promotion and life skills building. Information can also be handled well and disseminated through various media, such as instant messaging, Facebook, the Internet, smart phones, and other technology (see Andrea C. Bostrom: Technologic advances in psychiatric nursing: An update, in this issue). Psychiatric mental health nurses must be lifelong learners and stay abreast of the underpinnings of major SUDs, psychiatric disorders, and various drugs, both illicit and licit, particularly in their geographic region, as well as integrated evidence-based approaches to treat dual diagnoses.

## SUMMARY

Dual diagnosis is a prevalent and serious health problem. These disorders challenge psychiatric mental health and addiction nurses to treat 2 distinct disorders. Despite the advances in the treatment of these disorders, particularly integrated models of care, there remains a void in the ideal approach. This article offers psychiatric nurses opportunities to improve their expertise in the identification of vulnerable or high-risk populations by using integrated screening and brief interventions to discern treatment options. Patients who require comprehensive treatment to stabilize 1 or both disorders further challenge nurses to have a basic understanding of the powerful effects of substance use on psychiatric conditions and vice versa. Treatment approaches that have proven efficacy in the treatment of coexisting SUDs and psychiatric disorders are overviewed. Successful treatment outcomes are linked to individualized and person-centered approaches based on each patient's strengths, preferences, abilities and needs, and motivation to change. Equally important is for patients to have the education and support necessary for them to make decisions and participate in their treatment.

## REFERENCES

1. US Department of Health and Human Services, Substance Abuse and Mental Health Services Administration Center for Behavioral Health Statistics and Quality. 2010 National Survey on Drug Use and Health: Mental Health Findings. Available at: http://archive.samhsa.gov/data/NSDUH/2k10MH_Findings/2k10MH Results.htm#Ch4. Accessed November 27, 2015.
2. Hasin DS, Stinson PS, Ogburn E, et al. Prevalence, correlates, disability and co-morbidity of DSM-IV alcohol abuse and dependence in the United States: results from the National Epidemiologic Survey of Alcohol and Related Conditions. Arch Gen Psychiatry 2007;64:830–42.
3. Hasin DS, Grant BF. The epidemiologic survey of alcohol and related conditions (NESARC) waves 1 and 2: review and summary of findings. Soc Psychiatry Psychiatr Epidemiol 2015;50:1609–40.
4. Institute of Medicine (US) Committee on Crossing the Quality Chasm. Adaptation to mental health and addictive disorders. Improving the quality of health care for mental and substance-use conditions. Washington, DC: National Academies Press; 2006.
5. Crum RM, Mojtabaj R, Lazareck S, et al. A prospective assessment of reports of drinking to self-medicate mood symptoms with the incidence and persistence of alcohol dependence. JAMA Psychiatry 2013;70:718–26.
6. Robinson J, Sareen J, Cox BJ, et al. Role of self-medication in the development of comorbid anxiety and substance use disorders: a longitudinal investigation. Arch Gen Psychiatry 2011;68:800–7.
7. CDC Vital Signs. Prescription painkiller overdoses: a growing epidemic, especially among women. Atlanta (GA): US Department of Health and Human Services; 2013. Available at: www.cdc.gov/vitalsigns/prescriptionpainkilleroverdoses/index.html. Accessed December 2, 2015.
8. Rubinsky AD, Chen C, Batki SL, et al. Comparative utilization of pharmacotherapy for alcohol use disorder and other psychiatric disorders among U.S. Veterans Health Administration patients with dual diagnoses. J Psychiatr Res 2015;69: 150–7.
9. Shorter D, Hsieh J, Koston TR. Pharmacologic management of comorbid post-traumatic stress disorder and addictions. Am J Addict 2015;24:705–12.

10. Kelly TM, Daley DC, Douaihy AB. Treatment of substance abusing patients with comorbid psychiatric disorders. Addict Behav 2012;37:11–24.
11. Katz C, El-Gabalawy R, Keyes KM, et al. Risk factors for incident nonmedical prescription opioid use and abuse and dependence: results from a longitudinal nationally representative sample. Drug Alcohol Depend 2013;132:107–13.
12. US Preventive Services Task Force (USPSTF). Screening and behavioral counseling interventions in primary care to reduce alcohol misuse: U.S. Preventive Services Task Force recommendation statement. Ann Intern Med 2013;159: 210–8.
13. US Department of Health and Human Services, Substance Abuse and Mental Health Services Administration. Brief interventions and therapies for substance abuse KAP Keys for clinicians based on TIP 34. HHS publication no. (SMA) 153601. 2015. Available at: http://store.samhsa.gov/product/Brief-Interventions-and-Therapies-for-Substance-Abuse/BackInStock/SMA15-3601. Accessed December 3, 2015.
14. US Department of Health and Human Services. Substance abuse and mental health services administration. Treatment improvement protocol (TIP) series, no. 24: a guide to substance abuse services for primary care clinicians. Rockville (MD): SAMHSA/CSAT; 2008. Report No: (SMA) 97–3139. Available at: http://store.samhsa.gov/product/TIP-24-Guide-to-Substance-Abuse-Services-for-Primary-Care-Clinicians/SMA08-4075. Accessed December 6, 2015.
15. Ewing JA. Detecting alcoholism: the CAGE questionnaire. JAMA 1984;252: 1905–7.
16. Saunders JB, Aasland OG, Babor TF, et al. Development of Alcohol Use Disorders Identification Test (AUDIT): WHO Collaborative Project on Early Detection of Persons with Harmful Alcohol Consumption-II. Addiction 1993;88:791–804.
17. Miller WR, Rollnick S. Motivational interviewing: helping people change. 3rd edition. New York: Guilford Press; 2013.
18. National Institute on Drug Abuse; National Institutes of Health; US Department of Health and Human Services. DrugFacts: substance use in women. 2015. Available at: http://www.drugabuse.gov/publications/drugfacts/substance-use-in-women. Accessed December 5, 2015.
19. Torregrossa MM, Taylor JR. Learning to forget: manipulating extinction and reconsolidation processes to treat addiction. Psychopharmacology (Berl) 2013;226: 659–72.
20. American Psychiatric Association. Diagnostic and statistical manual of mental disorders: DSM-5. Washington, DC: American Psychiatric Association; 2013.
21. Farren CK, Snee L, Daly P, et al. Prognostic factors of 2-year outcomes of patients with comorbid bipolar disorder or depression with alcohol dependence: importance of early abstinence. Alcohol Alcohol 2013;48:93–8.
22. Farren CK, Murphy P, McElroy S. A 5-year follow-up of depressed and bipolar patients with alcohol use disorder in an Irish population. Alcohol Clin Exp Res 2014; 38:1049–58.
23. Jasinska AJ, Chen BT, Bonci A, et al. Dorsal medial prefrontal cortex (MPFC) circuitry in rodent models of cocaine use: implications for drug addiction therapies. Addict Biol 2015;20:215–26.
24. Murthy P, Chand P. Treatment of dual diagnosis disorders. Curr Opin Psychiatry 2012;25:194–200.
25. Milton AL, Schramm MJ, Wawrzynski JR, et al. Antagonism at NMDA receptors, but not β-adrenergic receptors, disrupts the reconsolidation of pavlovian conditioned approach and instrumental transfer for ethanol-associated conditioned stimuli. Psychopharmacology (Berl) 2012;219:751–61.

26. Barak S, Liu F, Ben Hamida S, et al. Disruption of alcohol-related memories by mTORC1 inhibition prevents relapse. Nat Neurosci 2013;16:1111–7.
27. McGovern MP, Lambert-Harris C, Xie H, et al. A randomized controlled trial of treatments for co-occurring substance use disorders and post-traumatic stress disorder. Addiction 2015;110:1194–204.
28. Antai-Otong D. Familial systems and family therapy. Biological and Behavioral Concepts of Psychiatric Mental Health Nursing. 2nd edition. Clifton Park (NY): Thomson Delmar Learning; p. 849–69.
29. Prochaska JO, DiClemente CC. The transtheoretical approach: crossing traditional boundaries of therapy. Homewood (IL): Dow Jones Irwin; 1984.

# Evidenced-Based Care of Adolescents and Families in Crisis

Cindy Parsons, DNP, ARNP, PMHNP-BC

## KEYWORDS

- Adolescent • Crisis • Crisis intervention • Family • Lethality assessment
- Risk and protective factors

## KEY POINTS

- Crises are precipitated by specific identifiable events and are determined by an individual's personal perception of the situation.
- Nurses regularly intervene with individuals and families in crisis across the continuum of care and in a wide variety of settings. The nursing process serves as the framework by which nurses assist those in crisis with a short-term solution-focused approach to crisis management.
- The Robert's Seven-Stage Crisis Intervention Model identifies key stages that individuals and families progress through as they attempt to solve the problem that precipitated crisis. The stages are sequential but may overlap as progress occurs.
- The first step in crisis intervention is the assessment of lethality (imminent danger of harm to self or others).
- Crisis intervention is a process in which a solution-focused approach is used to help the adolescent and their family to use their strengths and resources to develop and implement potential solutions to the problem at hand and return their family system to a state of equilibrium.

## INTRODUCTION

Life in the twenty-first century is rife with stress. Economic volatility, societal conflicts, traumatic events, political unrest, and terrorism are only a few of the serious stressors one may be exposed to. In addition to these stressors, individuals confront maturational and situational changes that contribute to stress. Generally, a person reacts and adapts to stress effectively; however, an unanticipated stressful situation can

This article is an update of an article previously published in *Nursing Clinics of North America*, Volume 38, Issue 1, March 2003.
Disclosure Statement: The author has no financial disclosures or conflict of interest to disclose.
Department of Nursing, University of Tampa, 401 West Kennedy Boulevard, Box 10 F, Tampa, FL 33606, USA
*E-mail address:* cindy.parsons@ut.edu

http://dx.doi.org/10.1016/j.cnur.2016.01.008
0029-6465/16/$ – see front matter © 2016 Elsevier Inc. All rights reserved.
nursing.theclinics.com

precipitate the evolution of a crisis. Adolescence is a time of rapid physical, emotional, and maturational change. It is a tumultuous time, because the teen is coping with a multitude of forces that will influence their transition from childhood to adulthood. Adolescence holds the potential for growth and maturation, but it can be a challenging and demanding time for the teen and their family. The addition of external stressors can tax the individual and family system, leading to crisis.

Crisis is a subjective reaction to a stressful life experience that so affects the stability of the individual that the ability to cope or function may be seriously compromised.[1] Crises are personal in nature, acute and not chronic, hold the potential for personal growth, and will resolve within a brief period of time. The available resources and ability to effectively use these will determine the outcome of the crisis. For those multi-stressed individuals and their families, the stresses of a particular circumstance may overwhelm their ability to use their resources, creating tension and escalating anxiety, which culminates in crisis.

This article provides an overview of germane points relative to the factors that contribute to the evolution and resolution of crises in adolescents and their families and the role of nurses in crisis intervention. It examines the categories of crisis, the risk factors that can potentiate, and protective factors that may mediate crisis for youth and their families. It further examines the role of nursing in identifying and working with families to implement strategies using a crisis intervention model that can help them return to an optimal level of functioning.

## CRISES

Crisis is not defined by the event or precipitant itself. Crisis is defined by the individual's perception and the extent of disruption of personal or familial homeostasis[2]; this leads to systemic disequilibrium that does not respond to protective factors, use of external support systems, or previously effective coping skills. Crisis threatens personal and family system organization but also offers great opportunities for growth and development. Crises are acute and time-limited and will be resolved one way or another within a brief period of time. Crises are categorized into the 3 following types:

A. *Situational Crises*—arising from external events that are unanticipated and perceived as a threat to the individual or family, for example, job loss, divorce, academic failure, or severe physical or mental illness.
B. *Maturational Crises*—occurs across the continuum of the life cycle. Each developmental stage is marked by tasks or goals marking the transition from one stage to the next. Disequilibrium is created as part of the maturational growth and development, creating greater vulnerability to crisis.
C. *Adventitious or Social Crises*—triggered by external events that are accidental, uncommon, and unanticipated, resulting in multiple losses and extraordinary environmental change. This type includes events such as tornadoes, flood, fire, terrorist attacks, or war.

Nurses work in a wide variety of health care settings and may be the first point of contact for the adolescent and their family challenged by the stressors that strain their current skills and resources and threaten to evolve into crisis.

## RISKS AND PROTECTIVE FACTORS

Understanding the risk and protective factors that mitigate the development of crisis within a family provides the nurse with a framework from which to implement intervention strategies. An understanding of these factors allows the nurse to view the patient and family from strength-based rather than a deficit-based perspective. A protective factor is "a characteristic at the biological, psychological, family or community level associated with a lower likelihood of problem outcomes or that reduces the negative impact of a risk factor on problem outcomes."[3]

Resilience is viewed as a key protective factor. It was originally thought of as an internal trait specific to the individual but now is viewed as a combination of individual and environmental and family system traits. Resilience is the capability of individuals, families, groups, and communities to understand and creatively draw on their internal and external strengths, resulting in effective coping with challenges and significant adversity in ways that promote health, wellness, and an increased ability to respond constructively to future adversity.[4,5] Protective factors are conditions in families and communities that when present improve the overall health and functioning of the adolescent and family. These factors serve as buffers assisting parents, who otherwise are at high risk for neglect or abuse of their child.

Protective factors, such as social connections, an understanding of child development, parenting skills, and strong family and social support, are identified as key in fostering the open communication and problem-solving that allow families to approach adverse circumstances as a learning experience and adapt.[6] Within the family, a supportive environment, individual empowerment, healthy boundaries, constructive use of time, positive values, and social competencies have been found to be strong protective factors that can mediate the outcomes of those identified as high-risk youth.[7] Peer influences can be categorized into either a risk or a protective factor. Support from prosocial peers in the home, school, or community can serve to protect a teen from violent or aggressive behavior within their environment or from the peer group.[8] Schools can also serve in a protective fashion. Schools that foster a healthy learning environment and positive adult and youth relationships tend to have fewer negative student behaviors, thereby creating a sense of safety and security.[9] In working with at-risk youth and their families, the nurse will assess and use the protective factors found within the family, peers, and schools to promote resilience and coping to intervene when risk factors threaten the family system.

Risk factors are ones that greatly increase the likelihood of a problem outcome. Adolescents as they traverse their developmental stage are more vulnerable to certain factors that increase the likelihood of disrupted individual or family system homeostasis. It is important for nurses who work with adolescents and their families to understand those that present the greatest risk and potentiate adverse outcomes.

## HIGH RISK FACTORS
### Mental Illness

According to current epidemiologic reports by the National Institutes of Health,[10] it is estimated that 21% of all youth aged 12 to 18 will or have experienced a seriously debilitating mental disorder. The most commonly diagnosed disorders were attention deficit hyperactivity disorder (ADHD), major depression, and autism spectrum disorder. In addition, schizophrenia and bipolar disorder are 2 serious and chronic psychiatric disorders with onset in the late teens to early twenties. Acute psychiatric illness can profoundly impact the lives of the individual and their family. The second leading cause of death in the adolescent population is suicide, with mood disorders being present in 80% of teens who attempt suicide. Young persons with psychiatric disorders have difficulty developing and maintaining interpersonal relationships, are more likely to perform poorly in academic and work settings, and are more likely to abuse illicit substances.[11]

## Sexuality

Teenage birth rates in the United States have declined significantly since the 1990s and are at the lowest documented rate in history. The teen birth rate for 2013 was 26.5 births per 1000 adolescents, down from 61.8 in 1991.[12] Despite this improvement, the nation is still a top leader of teenage pregnancies when compared with other industrialized nations. Teenagers who engage in unprotected sex are subject to unintended pregnancies and are at increased risk for contracting and spreading sexually transmitted infections (STIs). An unplanned pregnancy can result in crisis for the adolescent and family unit alike. Poor prenatal care and the copious stressors associated with teenage pregnancy may result in health complications for the mother and infant, interfere with access to education and employment, and ultimately prevent a young mother's ability to contribute to the immediate family unit and/or society as a whole.[13]

During adolescence, one of the most challenging yet important tasks that parents face is how to provide the structure and boundaries that helps a teen traverse the path from adolescence into adulthood. Testing limits, pushing boundaries, and trying on roles are many of the ways that the young person tries to build their identity during this journey. It is imperative that a parent understand what is testing and requires intervention or responsive limit-setting versus the adolescent being assertive about characteristics critical to their identify, such as sexual orientation or gender identity. Gender identity, sexual orientation, and comfort with oneself as a sexual being are key tasks of adolescence. There is controversy over whether gender identity is an inborn trait or learned and socialized role.[14] Starting at birth, children are socialized to familial and societal role expectations. New babies are dressed in pink or blue; toys are geared to the role of man or woman with sports toys for the boy and dolls for the girl. This trend continues into puberty, where social expectations and peer pressure may increase the expectation that one conform to gender expectations. Gender traits rarely fall exclusively into male or female traits but exist along a continuum with the individual having some characteristics of each. Gender identity and sexual orientation are not synonymous; being transgender is about identity, whereas being gay is about sexual orientation.[15] For the teen struggling with either of these complex issues, other forces, such as parental disapproval, rejection by friends and peers, and lack of a sufficient support system, can lead to anxiety, distress, low self-esteem, and depression.

Nurses in the primary care, school, or public health setting are often the first health care provider to have contact with the teen struggling with stressors related to sexual health, unintended pregnancy, or gender identity. Nurses working with these vulnerable adolescents need effective communication skills, active listening, empathy, and a supportive attitude to establish trust and develop a working relationship. The nurse provides support and guidance as she or he assists the young person to define the problem, explore their perspective, and understand its impact on their life. In working with minors, the nurse needs to have knowledge of the state and federal laws governing the reproductive rights of the individual and the role of parents or guardians in the decision-making process.

## Substance Use

A multitude of factors influence whether an adolescent uses alcohol or illicit substances, including the novelty of the experience, an attempt to cope with stress or problems, an attempt to improve academic performance, or simple peer pressure. Inherent in adolescence is the desire to seek new experiences and take risks as well as to carve out their own identity. Experimentation with illicit or prescription drugs may fulfill all of these normal developmental drives, but in an unhealthy way that can have very serious long-term consequences. Among the other factors influencing adolescent substance use is the availability of drugs within the neighborhood, community, and school and whether there is use by the adolescent's peer group.[16] The family environment is also important; violence, physical or emotional abuse, mental illness, or drug use in the household increases the likelihood an adolescent will use drugs. Finally, an adolescent's inherited genetic vulnerability; personality traits like poor impulse control or a high need for excitement; mental health conditions such as depression, anxiety, or ADHD; and beliefs such as that drug use is trendy and acceptable or harmless make it more likely that an adolescent will experiment with substance use.

Most teens do not escalate from experimentation or recreational use to developing an addiction or other substance use disorder. However, even experimentation is a problem. Drug use can be part of a pattern of risky behavior, including unsafe sex, driving while intoxicated, or other hazardous activities that increase the risk of serious injury. In teens with repetitive drug use, it can pose serious social and health risks,[17] including the following:

- School failure
- Interpersonal relationship problems with family, other adults, and peers
- Loss of interest in normal healthy activities
- Impaired memory
- Accidental injury
- Increased risk of STIs (like human immunodeficiency virus or hepatitis C)
- Mental illness
- Risk of unintentional death by overdose

### Technology and Media

Media and technology play a significant role in contemporary life, wielding influence on perceptions, interpersonal interactions, worldview, and understanding of the world. These influences can be positive or negative. On the positive side is the ability to rapidly access information, quickly learn of world events, interact with others near or far, and engage in recreational activities such as games or video viewing. A variety of tools allow people to be more productive and efficient with their time and academic or occupational performance. Negative influences can include the inappropriate portrayal of power, offensive language, and content of an explicit sexual and violent nature contained in many interactive games, television shows, and movies. Electronic media have become a much stronger influence on the adolescent's perspective of sexuality. Visual media often portray adult sexual encounters as casual and risk free, rarely including the risks of exposure to STIs and unintended pregnancy.

Another form of negative social interaction that has become increasingly prevalent is "cyberbullying." It has been defined as "covert, psychological bullying conveyed through electronic mediums."[18] Cyberbullying is an act of relational aggression, in which the perpetrator(s) attempt to cause psychological harm by damaging social relationships and degrading a person's social status. It can be carried out via cell phones, e-mails, Web sites, or social media that are commonly used for communication and interaction. Cyberbullying can lead to significant outcomes, such as emotional distress, anxiety, depressed mood, somatic illness, retaliatory violence, and even suicide.[19]

The Internet has revolutionized how everyone communicates and accesses information. Today's youth were born into a "wired" society and use electronic tools with comfort and ease. The dangers inherent in this ready access to social contacts and information from diverse sources, which may be reliable but can be informal and uncensored, are varied and often hidden. Parents may feel overwhelmed and challenged by their children's Internet capabilities and unsure of how to monitor, manage, and protect them from external influences.

## Violence

Although the overall rates of youth violence have declined since the 1990s, current trends in rates of interpersonal violence has reached epidemic proportions.[20] Youth violence is delineated as harmful behaviors that begin in childhood and can continue into early adulthood. It is the intentional use of physical force to threaten or inflict harm on another person, resulting in physical or emotional harm. This violence can affect a teen as a victim, witness, or perpetrator. Two of the leading causes of death in teens are homicide and suicide, resulting in approximately 6500 deaths annually.[20,21]

Domestic violence, including intimate partner violence, can have a disruptive and traumatic effect on a child who witnesses these acts. Studies have found these youth exhibit more aggressive and externalizing behavior, lower levels of social competence, and higher levels of depression and anxiety than their unaffected peers. Community violence is recognized as a major health problem that has far-reaching effects beyond the urban centers that it more commonly occurs in. Most public health efforts are focused on finding solutions for the causes and strengthening communities, while young persons who are exposed to and live in these communities become the direct or indirect victims of this violence. There are many types of community violence ranging from war, acts of terrorism, gang-related acts of violence, and bullying. The types of violence youth are exposed to become more aggressive and increase in severity as the child ages.[22]

Bullying is unwanted aggressive behavior among young people that involves a power imbalance and can be a one-time occurrence or repeated. It can take the form of physical or verbal threats, harassment, purposefully excluding someone from activities, or spreading rumors. Bullying can be direct and overt or more covert and subtle, involving social-emotional interactions such as gossip. It can take place in person, in verbal interactions, or through the use of electronic media or cyberbullying. The effects of bullying can be profound and affect the child emotionally, socially, and academically.

## Family

Over the course of the last half century, the state of the American family has been rapidly changing. Today, less than half of all children in the United States live in a traditional nuclear family. Today, family forms are complex and varied with the following types among those commonly found in American society: nuclear, single-parent, blended, unmarried biological, extended, and children living with grandparents or foster parents. Families are defined by reciprocal relationships in which persons are committed to one another.[23] Duvall[23] further identified core functions that were incumbent on the family system to meet the needs of individual members and its social role. What these functions are can depend on the societal norms, but key among these are to provide financial security, housing, and physical and emotional safety and security. Internal system influences on the health of families include family form, developmental stage, family lifestyle patterns, power structure, coping strategies, resilience, and connection to external supports. The level of family functioning, regardless of form, will greatly influence the members' abilities to individual and collectively manage societal and life stressors.

In Western society, individuality and freedom of choice are highly valued, yet each individual is molded and sustained by the interconnected web of human relationships, with the primary of these being the family. The dynamics of the family values, communication patterns, power structure roles, and boundaries significantly influence the beliefs and actions of individuals across and throughout the lifespan. The values and norms of the family significantly influence the beliefs and actions of the individual members. Healthy families can support and nurture one another and are flexible and adaptable in the face of stress or change, including developmental change. Multistressed families, such as those with a history of abuse or neglect, health problems, marital conflict, domestic or community violence, or financial stressors, may have a reduced capacity to cope effectively with stresses.[3] A healthy family provides its individual members with skills and tools to navigate functioning within the family, which can then be applied to interactions within the workplace, community, and society. These tools include communication skills, boundary delineation, emotional support, validation, and mutuality. Healthy families have permeable and flexible boundaries, clearly defined roles, and communication patterns. They are then better able to support and encourage one another in the face of change or stressful life events.

## CRISIS INTERVENTION

Contemporary crisis theory was first proposed by Lindemann,[24] who strongly believed that preventive measures, when implemented with those suffering acute grief, could eliminate the psychological disorganization and distress associated with the severe anxiety of grief. Caplan[1] further refined the theory and developed strategies for crisis intervention. As advanced practice psychiatric nursing evolved, Aquilera and Messick[2] further refined the crisis intervention model (**Fig. 1**), and its applicability to nurses working in the specialty of mental health. This model could be applied to individuals, families, and groups and identified crisis recovery factors and individual and system resources that should be sued to resolve crises. Aquilera and Messick[2] noted that the equilibrium of persons in crisis is significantly affected by 3 factors, their

- Perception of the problem
- Support system
- Coping mechanisms

They proposed that balancing the risk and protective factors would stabilize the system and restore equilibrium.

Roberts'[25,26] in conceptualizing the process of crisis intervention, identified 7 key stages that those in crisis must progress through. These stages should proceed sequentially, but may overlap and are essential for the progression from crisis to resolution. In applying this model (**Fig. 2**) effectively, the nurse will need to assess and gauge where those affected are in terms of stage and goal attainment. The stages should serve as a guide for progression and not a rigid frame to be so tightly adhered to so as to interfere with the individuality and use of resources by those in crisis. The use of this model can facilitate the nurse's intervening by maintaining the focus of care on the rapid assessment of the client's perceived problem, developing a therapeutic alliance and working relationship to implementation of strategies and resolution of the acute crisis. The use of an evidence-based model allows nurses of all specialties and depth of experience to effectively work with individuals, families, groups, and communities affected by crisis.

## CRISIS INTERVENTION, THE NURSING PROCESS, AND ROBERT'S SEVEN-STAGE MODEL

All crisis intervention models begin with a thorough assessment before initiating any intervention strategies. This first stage in the Robert's model[25] addresses a key risk

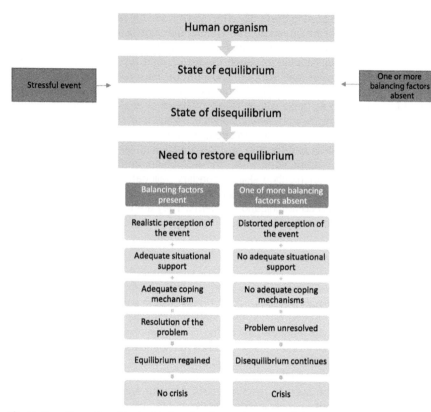

**Fig. 1.** Paradigm: the effect of balancing factors in a stressful event.

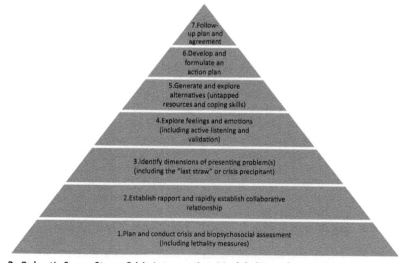

**Fig. 2.** Robert's Seven-Stage Crisis Intervention Model. (*Data from* Roberts AR, Ottens AJ. The seven-stage crisis intervention model: a road map to goal attainment, problem solving and crisis resolution. Oxford Journals, Medicine 2005;5(4);329–39.)

factor: before engaging people in crisis intervention, it is important to assure the safety of those involved and allow the focus of care to be on crisis resolution.

## Assessment

### Stage 1: assessing lethality
As the nurse establishes a formal relationship with the adolescent and family, he or she must determine whether any of the individuals pose a significant risk of harm to self or others. Suicide is one of the leading causes of death in the teen population, and suicide assessment is a core mental health nursing competency. Thorough assessment includes assessment of ideation, intent, plan, and access to lethal means. The SAFE-T (Suicide Assessment Five-Step Evaluation and Triage) assessment[27] assists the nurse in determining a level of risk and probability of a suicide attempt and provides guidance in developing a plan of interventions appropriate for the individual. The first step is to perform the assessment and identify risk factors with special emphasis on those that can be modified to reduce risk. Next, identify protective factors noting those that can be enhanced to reduce risk. The third step is direct inquiry about the individual's intent to commit suicide. Finally, these are categorized, and a level of risk is determined. For those at high risk, treatment and amelioration of suicidality, which may include hospitalization, are imperative before implementing crisis intervention. The final step in this assessment involves thorough documentation of the assessment, interventions, and outcomes. Ensuring the safety of those involved provides a solid foundation from which to move forward and continue crisis intervention.

### Stage 2: establishing rapport and communication
Developing the therapeutic relationship and a sense of trust is key to effective communication. Developing rapport is more than ease of conversation; it involves clarifying roles and boundaries, building trust, and acquiring an empathic understanding of the patients' suffering. Kanel[28] identifies 5 key attending skills that promote the development of rapport. These skills include attending behaviors (verbal and nonverbal), a supportive questioning style, paraphrasing or reframing, reflection of feelings, and summarizing. Listening to and responding appropriately to the client's perception and story further the rapport and engagement of the adolescent and family.

### Stage 3: identifying major problems
The core task of this stage is to assist the patient and family to define the problem using their perceptual lens. Although it requires time, the nurse should interview each family member individually and then bring the family together as a whole to define the problem. As they convey their story, the nurse uses clarifying questions to assist in prioritizing problems and identifying actions already taken in an attempt to solve the problem. Eliciting information about unsuccessful attempts may allow those involved to be open to alternative approaches and solutions. Using a solutions-focused approach, the nurse focuses on the strengths, resources, and capacities of the individuals, enhancing the trust and rapport essential for a successful nurse-patient relationship. Once the problem has been defined as clearly as possible, the nurse will help the clients define their outcome goal or goals. This stage requires skill and adept communication because clients can get stuck in airing their feelings and will need guidance and support to stay focused on problem and goal definition.

### Stage 4: dealing with feelings and emotions
Inherent in this stage is therapeutic use of self. The nurse facilitates expression of emotions and feelings while maintain a solution-focused approach. Nurses are human beings, and as such, have values, beliefs, and opinions. One of the most difficult aspects

of caring for those experiencing distress and disequilibrium is maintaining therapeutic neutrality. By using therapeutic communication skills, such as active listening, empathy, and rephrasing, the nurse can help the individual and family to clarify their thoughts, feelings, and expectations. In addition, the nurse may be able to de-escalate tension by asking clarifying questions or paraphrasing statements that initially were negatively interpreted and perceived. Effective management of emotions and creating a calm influence and stability within the system then allows for the transition to generating solutions.

### Planning

### Stage 5: explore and generate alternatives

As the therapeutic alliance evolves and strengthens, crisis intervention moves into the problem-solving phase. In working with adolescents and their families, the nurse needs to be cognizant of the cognitive and developmental differences between teens and adults. Adults have had more experience with problem-solving; however, the best solution for the current crisis may come from the adolescent or be a compilation of ideas generated by all. Problem-solving or task-centered approaches can prevent unclear, unfocused crisis intervention. Remaining solution-focused, the nurse helps the family members create and discuss alternatives, integrating previously identified strengths and capacities. Exploration of previously used successful coping strategies may help them remember what worked and what elements of the approach facilitated a positive outcome. As anxiety and tension levels are typically elevated during crisis, it may be useful to have individuals write out their thoughts and proposed solutions and then discuss the usefulness or appropriateness of each.

### Implementation

### Stage 6: formulating an action plan

Creating an action plan is a 2-step process. The first step includes the solution generating that occurs in stage 5. As the nurse facilitates solution generation, he or she must guide the clients to develop an action plan implementing these solutions. The nurse must also work with the family so they develop an agreed on outcome and have a clear understanding of what is needed to bring resolution to the current state of distress. In the second step, the nurse works with the adolescent and family to assure that the action plan is realistic and feasible and will help to achieve the desired outcome. Do they have the resources to enact the plan? Do they need additional resources? Can the plan be implemented without causing further significant disruption? Who is leading the change? If the agreed on plan does not yield the desired outcome, when will they enact alternate strategies?

The goal of crisis intervention is to resolve the current problem stressing the system and creating disequilibrium. As the crisis resolves, the individuals and family system should return to a precrisis or higher level of functioning and not a regressed level.

### Evaluation

### Stage 7: termination and follow-up

During termination, the primary goal is for the individuals to evaluate their progress and consolidate the actions that led to crisis resolution and improved functionality. The nurse should promote celebration of their successes and help each to recognize their positive contribution to the change. The adolescent and their family should take credit for their ability to use their strengths and combined resources to generate solutions, implement change, and effectively return their family system to a fully functional state. In addition to providing this positive feedback, the nurse begins the process of termination. In conjunction with the family, the nurse sets an after-intervention follow-up visit (usually 2 to 3 weeks later) to evaluate the after-crisis status of those involved. The nurse provides clear communication that the family will have access to the nurse but is responsible for continuing their progress and resumption of their normal daily life. The process of closure helps the clients to maintain a future-oriented view and not focus on the stresses of the immediate past and crisis.

## SUMMARY

Contemporary life poses many challenges, with people being exposed to unpredictable and often traumatic stressors. Throughout the maturational process from childhood to adulthood, adolescents face additional risks that can create additional stress or tax the resources of the teen and their family to the point of crisis. During crisis, the normal means of coping with stress is ineffective and the anxiety and tension intolerable, disrupting the normal balance of the family system. Crisis by its very nature is acute and time-limited, requiring focused and targeted intervention to help the individual and family return to their previous or even an improved functional state. Nurses work with teens in a wide variety of settings and are optimally suited to provide intervention to those in crisis.

Crisis intervention is a brief solution-focused approach the focuses on the clients' strengths to resolve crises. The Robert's Seven-Stage Crisis Intervention Model provides an evidence-based approach to crisis intervention and a useful framework from which to evaluate the progress of those involved. During the initial contact with the adolescent and their family, the nurse performs a lethality assessment. Once the risk of harm is mitigated, the nurse can then work with the clients to generate solutions to the perceived problem and use their strengths and resources to return the system to the equilibrium disrupted by the crisis.

## REFERENCES

1. Caplan G. Preventative psychiatry. New York: Basic books; 1964.
2. Aquilera D, Messick J. Crisis intervention theory and methodology. 1st edition. St Louis (MO): C.V. Mosby; 1970.
3. Benzies K, Mychasiuk R. Fostering family resilience: a review of the key protective factors. Child Fam Soc Work 2008;14:103–14.
4. Donnon T, Hammond W. A psychometric assessment of self-reported youth resilience: Assessing the Developmental Strengths questionnaire. Psychol Rep 2007; 100(3 Pt 1):963–78.
5. O'Connell ME, Boat T, Warner KE. Preventing mental, emotional, and behavioral disorders among young people: progress and possibilities. Washington, DC: The National Academies Press; and U.S. Department of Health and Human Services, Substance Abuse and Mental Health Services Administration; 2009.
6. Garfat T, Van Bockern S. Families and the circle of courage. Reclaiming Children and Youth 2010;8(4):4–37.
7. Chew W, Osseck J, Raygor D, et al. Developmental assets of youth in a juvenile justice facility. J Sch Health 2010;80(2):66–72.
8. Aisenberg E, Herrenkohl T. Community violence in context: risk and resilience in children and families. J Interpers Violence 2008;23:296–316.
9. Powers JD, Bowen GL, Rose RA. Using social environmental assets to identify intervention strategies for promoting school success. Child Schools 2005;27: 177–87.
10. National Institutes of Health. Any mental illness (AMI) among adults. 2013. Available at: http://www.nimh.nih.gov/health/statistics/prevalence/any-mental-illness-ami-among-adults.shtml. Accessed November 17, 2015.

11. Merikangas KR, He JP, Burstein M, et al. Lifetime prevalence of mental disorders in U.S. adolescents: results from the National Comorbidity Study-Adolescent Supplement (NCS-A). J Am Acad Child Adolesc Psychiatry 2010;49(10):980–9.
12. Martin JA, Hamilton BE, Osterman MJK, et al. Births: final data for 2013. Hyatts-ville (MD): National Center for Health Statistics; 2015.
13. Hoffman SD. Kids having kids: economic and social consequences of teen preg-nancy. Washington, DC: The Urban Institute Press; 2008.
14. Steensma TD, Kreukel BP, deVries AL, et al. Gender identity development in adolescence. Horm Behav 2013;64(2):288–97.
15. Simonelli C, Rossi R, Tripodi MF, et al. Gender identity disorder and pre-adolescence: a pilot study. Sexologies 2006;16:22–8.
16. Substance Abuse & Mental Health Services Administration. Results from the 2013 National Survey on Drug Use and Health. Summary of national findings. Rockville (MD): SAMSHA; 2014. HHS publication # (SMA) 14-4887.
17. Johnston LD, O'Malley PM, Bachman JG, et al. Monitoring the future: national sur-vey results on drug use, 1975-2010. Vol. 1, Secondary school students. Ann Ar-bor (MI): The Institute for Social Research, The University of Michigan; 2011.
18. Shariff S, Gouin R. Cyber-dilemmas: gendered hierarchies, free expression and cyber safety in schools. In: Leach F, Mitchell C, editors. Safety and security in a networked world: balancing cyber rights and responsibilities. Oxford (United Kingdom): Oxford University Press; 2005. p. 11–20.
19. Carter J, Wilson FL. Cyberbullying: a 21st century health care phenomenon. Pe-diatr Nurs 2015;41(3):115–27.
20. Centers for Disease control and Prevention. Youth risk behavior surveillance—United States, 2011. MMWR Surveill Summ 2012;61(4):1–162.
21. Centers for Disease Control and Prevention. Homicide rates among persons aged 10-24-years-old United States, 1081-2010. 2013. Available at: www.cdc.gov/mmwr/preview/mmwrhtml/mm6227.htm. Accessed November 27, 2015.
22. Finkelhor D, Turner H, Ormrod R, et al. Violence, abuse, and crime exposure in a national sample of children and youth. Pediatrics 2009;124(5):1411–23.
23. Duvall E. Family development. Oxford (United Kingdom): J.P. Lipincott; 1957.
24. Lindemann E. Symptomatology and management of acute grief. Am J Psychiatry 1944;101:141–8.
25. Roberts A. An overview of crisis theory and crisis intervention. In: Roberts A, ed-itor. Crisis intervention handbook. 2nd edition. New York: Oxford University Press; 2000.
26. Roberts AR, Ottens AJ. The seven-stage crisis intervention model: a road map to goal attainment, problem solving and crisis resolution. Oxford Journals, Medicine 2005;5(4):329–39.
27. Suicide Prevention Resource Center. Suicide Assessment Five-Step Evaluation and Triage for mental health professionals. SAFE-T. 2008. Available at: http://www.sprc.org/sectionIII/suicideassessmentfive-step-evaluation-and-triage-safe-t. Accessed November 27, 2015.
28. Kanel K. A guide to crisis intervention. 5th edition. Belmont (CA): Cengage Learning; 2013.

# Managing the Care of the Older Patient with Delirium and Dementia

Carolyn Seeganna, MS, RN, CNS, ANP[a],*,
Deborah Antai-Otong, MS, APRN, PMHCNS-BC, FAAN[b]

## KEYWORDS

- Geriatric psychiatric emergencies • Delirium • Dementia • Cognitive disorders

## KEY POINTS

- Nurses are on the frontline of health care and can identify symptoms that assist in distinguishing symptoms or delirium and dementia and provide appropriate interventions.
- Delirium and dementia pose serious human and financial burdens, including morbidity/mortality, lengthened hospitalizations, increased staff demands, safety deficits, and decline in patient and caregiver quality of life.
- Efforts to facilitate health resolution and restore the patient and caregivers to an optimal level of functioning must be priorities.

Nearly 45 million or 1 of every 7 Americans are aged 65 or older,[1] with more than 23% in fair or poor health, and more than 20% making 10 or more health care visits per year.[2] Only a small percentage of older adults seek care complaining of emotional distress. Older adults are more likely to seek health care for physical complaints rather than psychiatric problems, subsequently challenging nurses in vast clinical settings to distinguish medical conditions from underlying psychiatric conditions and initiating appropriate interventions. Because nurses are often on the frontline of health care and are able to establish rapport with their patients, they are in fortuitous position to intervene when older adults present with medical and psychiatric conditions to reduce their potential negative outcomes.

This article is an update of an article previously published in *Nursing Clinics of North America*, Volume 38, Issue 1, March 2003.
Disclosure Statement: The authors have nothing to disclose.
[a] US Department of Veterans Affairs, Mat-Su Community Based Outpatient Clinic, 865 North Seward Meridian Parkway, Wasilla, AK 99654, USA; [b] Department of Veterans Affairs, Veterans Integrated Service Networks-(VISN-17), 2301 E. Lamar Boulevard, Arlington, TX 76006, USA
* Corresponding author.
*E-mail address:* Carolyn.Seeganna@va.gov

Of particular importance to nurses is identifying symptoms that assist in distinguishing symptoms of delirium and dementia and providing appropriate interventions. Patients with delirium or dementia often are brought in by family members or friends who are concerned about their acute or progressive confusion, cognitive impairment, and subsequent deteriorating level of functioning and dependency on others. Although delirium and dementias are medical conditions, these clients often are brought into primary care and mental health treatment centers because of their behavioral problems and risk of violence toward self and others. Efforts to discern underlying causes, treatment approaches, and dispositions challenge nurses in various settings to understand the patient's mental status changes and cognitive deficits.

## PREVALENCE AND COST OF COGNITIVE DISORDERS

Delirium and other cognitive disorders are common, costly, and morbid, particularly among older adults. Delirium is a medical emergency that requires immediate evaluation and management to reduce its potential negative sequelae. Nurses are in pivotal, frontline positions to enable them to recognize high-risk older adults and initiate interventions that promote healthy outcomes for the patient presenting with delirium and various dementias.

## DELIRIUM

Delirium is a prevalent complication of acute medical conditions, particularly in older adults. In the general population, 1% to 2% of people aged 65 and older have delirium,[3] but rates increase with age, with delirium occurring in up to 14% of people greater than age 85.[4] Delirium occurs in 10% to 30% of geriatric patients in emergency departments,[5] and in more than 60% of nursing home residents.[4] Contributing factors include systemic disorders, such as infection, metabolic disturbances, and adverse drug reactions. Delirium occurs in about 32% of intensive care unit patients[6] and between 5% and 50% of geriatric postoperative patients.[7] Postsurgical delirium often arises from the demands of surgery on physiologic functioning, such as sleep disturbances, immobilization, presence of urinary catheter, or inadequately controlled pain. Delirium increases risks of complications like hospital-acquired infections and pressure ulcers, prolongs hospitalization by up to 8 days, and carries twice the 12-month mortality of patients without delirium.[4,8,9] These data suggest that delirium increases the risk of cognitive and functional decline and mortality after hospitalization compared with nondelirious states. These findings are consistent with those of other researchers, who state that the course of delirium is not easily resolved and symptoms may persist longer than hospitalization or treatment in various clinical settings.[10] Although delirium can occur at any age, older adults, especially those with pre-existing dementia and other neurologic conditions, are at a greater risk. A key to early identification and management of delirium involves prevention. By understanding delirium, identifying predisposition risk factors, and ultimately managing delirium, nurses can reduce the potentially deleterious consequences.

### Definition and Clinical Features

Delirium is a complex, potentially reversible neuropsychiatric disorder characterized by fluctuating disturbances in attention, awareness, and cognition that develops over hours or days and represents a change in baseline.[11] Historically, delirium was considered transient, with recovery expected once the triggering underlying medical condition resolved.[12] However, delirium is now recognized as multifaceted, persistent interactions of multiple predisposing and precipitating factors common in geriatric populations, such as comorbidity, polypharmacy, metabolic disturbances, and infections.[13] Persistent cognitive deficits also have been linked to a comorbid dementing condition that was exposed by the delirious state. Delirium is often unrecognized and misdiagnosed in older adults.[3,14] Findings from follow-up visits indicate that delirium has a persistent course and that failure to respond to treatment during hospitalization increases this risk.[12] Typically, clients with delirium exhibit disorientation, mood disturbance, inattention, altered sleep/wake cycles, disorganized behaviors, and perceptual disturbances.[4] Usually, these symptoms are worse during the evening, resulting in sun-downing syndrome manifested by marked confusion and behavioral disturbances that may lead to serious injury. Data from caregivers or significant others often reveal symptoms that emerge over hours or days (rapid onset) and a waxing and waning course. A caregiver may describe the patient as being "like himself" 1 minute and the next "he acted like a wild man."

The Confusion Assessment Method (CAM)[15] targets 5 general criteria that assist in the diagnosis of delirium:

- Rapid or acute onset (change in mental status)
- Fluctuating course
- Inattention
- Disorganized
- Alterations in consciousness.

This instrument's focus is on the clinical rather than causative features of the syndrome, often revealing relevant data, such as:

- When did you notice changes in the patient's behavior?
- Do the symptoms change during the course of the day or night?
- Have you noticed if the patient has difficulty focusing or maintaining attention?
- Does the patient have rambling, irrelevant, or incoherent speech or lack logic to his or her flow of ideas?
- Have you noticed any changes in the patient's level of consciousness (eg, drowsy, easily startled, and difficult to wake up)?

Although the CAM remains the gold standard for bedside delirium assessment, critics cite the need for substantial interviewer training, required cognitive assessment, variations in clinical applications, and challenges applying the tool in general medical settings.[16] The newer 3-D CAM offers a streamlined assessment with benefits, including simplified completion without need for extensive training or certain administrator clinical licensure.[17]

Many patients with delirium may have symptom subtypes classified as hyperactive (30%) (hallucinations, repetitive behaviors, aggression, and delusions) or hypoactive (25%) (lethargic, quiet, withdrawn), but most (45%) fluctuate within a mixed spectrum of hyperactive and hypoactive subtypes with periods of lucidity in between.[4,18,19] Data from an empirical study of delirium subtypes indicate that hypoactive subtypes have the poorest mortality rates yet are least likely to be accurately assessed.[20,21] Several psychiatric disorders may mimic symptoms delirium symptoms, such as apathy and fatigue in depression and hypoactive delirium and hallucinations and delusions in schizophrenia and hyperactive delirium. However, only delirious patients have accompanying altered level of consciousness or cognitive impairment with acute onset over hours or days and/or fluctuation over the course of a day.[22] Other symptoms, such as urinary incontinence, emotional lability (eg, rage, anger, fear, apathy), shakiness or tremors, uncooperativeness, treatment or food refusal, wandering, and concurrent dementia, further complicate the assessment process, and an estimated 30% to 60% of all deliriums go undiagnosed.[19]

It is essential to assess for premorbid histories of personality changes, impaired judgment, restlessness, anxiety, fear, irritability, and incoherence that precede changes in their level of consciousness, which are often unrecognized by health care providers. It is also important to know the patient's baseline mental status. These patients tend to be poor historians, making it necessary to obtain data from other sources. Family members or caregivers offer important information about the patient's baseline level of functioning and can assist in making a diagnosis of delirium. Because of the potential deleterious course of delirium, which previously was thought to be transient, nurses in various clinical settings, including primary care, extended care facilities, and postoperative and medical-surgical units, must identify older patients as high-risk patients and work with an interdisciplinary team to reduce the incidence of delirium and ultimately improve overall health outcomes.

### Causative Factors

As previously mentioned, delirium is likely to arise from an underlying acute medical condition, such as metabolic disturbances, fluid and electrolyte imbalance, renal failure, neurologic disorders such as stroke, and adverse drug reactions. Scientists state that these medical conditions affect the ascending reticular activating system that is manifested as attention and concentration and sleep-wake cycle deficits and changes in sensorium.[23] The ascending reticular activating system is involved in modulating the level of consciousness. The precise severity and course of delirium are complex but often are influenced by the patient's present medical and mental status, underlying general medical conditions, or drug toxicity that insults cerebral metabolism and biochemical processes, particularly in the dopamine and γ-aminobutyric acid pathways. Others hypothesize that impairment of central cholinergic transmission supports the manifestation of symptoms associated with anticholinergic toxicity.[19,24] The use of various medications with anticholinergic properties contribute to delirium in older adults. Examples of these are anticholinergic agents (benztropine), high-dose antipsychotics (olanzapine, risperidone), narcotics (meperidine), antihistamines (diphenhydramine), long-acting benzodiazepines (diazepam), ranitidine, and antidepressants like selective serotonin reuptake inhibitors (fluoxetine), and tricyclics (amitriptyline).[24,25]

Numerous medical conditions can cause delirium, including infections, intoxication and withdrawal syndromes, retention problems, structural insults, and hypoxic conditions. Polypharmacy, various medications, and toxins also can produce delirium. Hospitalized residents from extended care facilities are especially vulnerable to conditions that increase the risk of delirium, including advanced age, pre-existing neurologic conditions, sensory deficits, polypharmacy, and poor functional status.[26]

Inouye and Charpentier[27] developed a predictive model for delirium based on 5 independent precipitating factors, as follows:

- The use of physical restraints
- Impaired nutritional status
- Polypharmacy or more than 3 medications added
- The use of a bladder catheter

These data also indicate that each precipitating factor occurred more than 24 hours before the onset of delirium. Additional precipitating factors include acute cardiac or pulmonary events, infections such as respiratory and urinary tract infections, fecal impaction, fluid or electrolyte disturbances, urinary retention anemia, and uncontrolled pain.[28] Nurses can consider these predictive factors to enhance the identification of high-risk older adults in diverse clinical settings and reduce the potentially deleterious courses of this acute medical condition.

### Acute Management

The presence of delirium is a solemn diagnostic sign in older adults because there is a 10-fold higher death occurrence in hospitalized delirious patients, impaired physical and cognitive recovery rates, and increased risk of hospital-acquired infection, falls, pressure ulcers, and incontinence.[4,28,29] The optimal goal of delirium is prevention, early identification, and appropriate management of this acute confusion state. Because of the complexity of delirium, nurses, other health care providers, and family members must play active roles in assessing the patient's symptoms and identifying the primary condition causing delirium. This process begins with establishing rapport with the patient and significant others. If the patient is exhibiting signs of violence and marked agitation, safety must be a priority. Safety measures must include determining the level of dangerousness to self and others, gathering data about past violence, and using measures that reduce agitation and confusion. Approaching the patient cautiously but respectfully and introducing oneself, orientating the patient, and anticipating the patient's anxiety enable the nurse to assess the patient's behavior further.

### Assessment and Diagnosis

A comprehensive physical and psychosocial assessment is a vital part of the differential diagnosis that involves an interdisciplinary approach. Perhaps the most challenging aspect of assessing the patient with delirium is not the diagnosis, but the identification and correction of the underlying medical condition.[19,26] The data-gathering process involves making a differential diagnosis of medical and psychiatric conditions, such as depression, psychotic disorders, and dementia. Information concerning substance abuse and medication review, including recent additions, changes in dose and discontinuation, and prescribed and over-the-counter drugs, is crucial to making a differential diagnosis. Because medications and polypharmacy have been linked to delirium, this must be ruled out during this process. The Mini Mental State Examination (MMSE) is a widely used screening tool that measures the degree of cognitive deficits and helps quantify the severity of symptoms.[30] The MMSE can produce high false-positive rates in older adults who have less than an eighth-grade education and who are not fluent in English. The physical examination needs to focus on ruling out infection, cardiovascular abnormalities, urinary retention, and fecal impaction. Laboratory studies, including a chemistry profile, complete blood count with differential, thyroid function, vitamin B12, urinalysis, toxicology screens, electrocardiogram, chest film, blood urea nitrogen, and oxygen saturation, are useful in making a differential diagnosis.

### Interventions

Major treatment goals involve reducing complications inherent with hospitalization, correcting the underlying medical condition, mitigating causative factors, ensuring safety, and supporting patient and family integrity. Successful treatment planning of delirium requires an interdisciplinary approach.

The management of delirium also includes supporting physiologic, psychosocial, and environmental function and integrity. Supporting physiologic integrity involves correcting underlying medical conditions, such as fluid and electrolyte imbalance, with appropriate measures and monitoring mental and physical status. Physiologic support also may include pharmacologic interventions that reduce delusions and hallucinations and agitation and irritability. Prophylactic antipsychotics shorten duration and decrease severity of dementia symptoms in at-risk perioperative patients and may even help prevent delirium altogether.[31–33] Haloperidol has a variety of formulations providing valuable administration options of administration barriers like agitation and psychosis, with onset of action within 30 minutes, with available readministration every 30 minutes as needed for agitation and other acute symptom containment, although daily doses exceeding 4.5 mg daily were associated with increased extrapyramidal symptoms (EPS) and should likely be avoided in older adults with parkinsonism.[26] Compared with typical antipsychotics, second-generation agents (SGA) like olanzapine, quetiapine, or risperidone have increased anticholinergic, hypotensive, and sedation side-effect risks as well as fewer administration choices, such as no intravenous formulations.[24] However, SGA have comparable efficacy without EPS likelihood and are increasingly becoming first-line medication choices.[31,34,35] Benzodiazepines should be avoided in older adults because of side effects that further impair cognitive function and produce drowsiness and disinhibition. Care must be taken to avoid sedation, and restraints must be avoided when possible to maintain safety and reduce complications. All of these side effects increase the risk of injuries resulting from falls and aggressive behaviors.

Psychosocial support involves introducing oneself, providing orientation, explaining procedures, monitoring mental status change, and ensuring the patient is never left alone. Throughout the assessment and treatment process, family members are an integral part of the treatment team. Nurses must provide health education and reassurance to the family members that delirium is normally reversible and often improves over time. It is also important to point out that some patients' symptoms persist for weeks to months. Families also must be instructed to improve the patient's mental and physical health by avoiding polypharmacy, providing adequate hydration and nutrition, and reporting worsening symptoms. Environmental support involves securing safety; reducing stimuli such as loud noises and too many people in the room; maintaining a well-lit room to ensure sensory and perceptual integrity; minimizing sleep disruptions; and ensuring that self-care needs like toileting are met.[13,26]

### Evaluation

A return to a previous level of physical and mental functioning is a criterion for measuring the outcome of treatment approaches. Positive outcomes generally reflect an accurate diagnosis and correction of the underlying medical condition.

Overall, delirium is a common medical condition characterized by attention and sensorium disturbances developing over a short period. This potentially fatal disorder parallels underlying physiologic consequences of a general medical condition and most commonly is found in older adults. Patients presenting with acute confused states or alterations in sensorium or cognitive function must be assessed quickly to rule out delirium and to initiate appropriate interventions to correct the underlying medical condition. Exceptional nursing care seems to be crucial to successful prevention and treatment of delirium. Nurses are on the frontline of health care and are in a prime position to assess these patients and collaborate with other health care providers to reduce the potentially negative outcome of delirium and return the patient to a previous or higher level of mental and physical functioning.

## DEMENTIA

The 5th edition of the *Diagnostic and Statistical Manual* retired "dementia" in favor of major neurocognitive disorder. However, dementia is still acceptable for use in etiologic subtypes where the term is standard and is the diagnostic descriptor used in this article.[11]

Dementia, similar to delirium, is a clinical syndrome characterized by acquired losses of cognitive and emotional abilities that interfere with the patient's level of functioning and quality of life. Up to 5 million Americans had Alzheimer-type dementia in 2013, and by 2050, that number is expected to reach 14 million.[36] A preponderance of evidence indicates that the incidence of dementia, both senile and vascular types, increases with age, with incidences of all-cause dementia doubling every 5 years after age 65, with incidence rates up to 41% of people aged 100 and older.[37] Dementia increases the risk of psychotic behaviors, such as hallucinations, especially visual and tactile forms; delusions and illusions; and behavioral disturbances, during the course of illness.[38] For the purposes of this article, Alzheimer disease (AD), an irreversible dementia, is the prototype of dementia, and the focus is on interventions to manage psychosis and behavioral disturbances. One study found that 97% of clients with dementia experience at least one neuropsychiatric disturbance sometime during the course of their illness, most commonly apathy, depression, and delusions but also disinhibition and elation.[39,40]

### Definition and Clinical Features

Progressive dementias, such as AD, in contrast to delirium, which has a rapid or acute onset, have an insidious onset and progressive course beginning with short-term memory loss that eventually results in substantial global deterioration of mental and physical function. Clinical features of dementia reflect the underlying degenerative processes in brain regions affecting cognition, evidenced by significant decline in one or more the following domains[41,42]:

- Complex attention (difficulty sustaining attention during competing stimuli like concurrent conversation and television; unable to perform multiple simultaneous tasks like finger tapping and reading)
- Executive function (difficulty with multistep tasks that require independent decision-making, problem-solving, and sequencing like paying bills and household chores)
- Learning and memory (repetitive questions and difficulty tracking conversations; requires prompting to stay on task; forgetting events or appointments; getting lost on a familiar route)
- Language (difficulty recalling common words while speaking; echolalia; forgetting names of family and friends)
- Perceptual-motor (difficulties with previously familiar activities like driving, dressing, using a telephone; "sundowners" confusion and disorientation with fading light)
- Social cognition (decreased sensitivity to social cues and needs of others; impaired reasoning such as not appreciating risks of going outdoors in poor weather while in nightclothes; poor insight)

Memory deficits are gradual and often represent a prominent early symptom of dementia. Typically the patient has difficulty learning new information and is forgetful (cannot remember where the keys are). Other patients have difficulty recognizing loved ones and common objects, such as a pen or watch, and have problems getting lost in familiar neighborhoods. Their judgment is impaired, and their ability to calculate or engage in abstract reasoning progressively declines.[11]

### Causative Factors

The exact cause of neurodegenerative changes of AD is obscure, but genetics, familial vulnerability, and advanced age have been identified as contributing factors. Most postmortem studies reveal alterations in neuroanatomic structures and neurobiochemical processes. AD, similar to other progressive neurocognitive disorders, has a degenerative course that involves neurofibrillary tangles in the cerebral cortex and accumulation of β-amyloid plaques in the nucleus basalis of Meynert synapses.[43] The hippocampus, which is housed in the medial temporal lobe, and the amygdala are essential for the formation and storage of immediate and recent memories and their relevance. The neocortex region of the brain involves higher brain or executive function, specifically neuroanatomic processes related to language and intelligence. Initially the parietal and temporal lobes are affected and later the frontal lobes. Personality changes, such as depression or distrust, are associated with frontal lobe destruction. This progressive destruction accounts for early symptoms of AD and subsequent global cognitive decline.

Destruction of diverse brain regions results in an inability to store, retrieve, and learn new information, ultimately affecting the ability to recognize common objects (anomia) and loved ones (agnosia). Destruction to the cortex primarily involves the parietal and temporal lobes, leading to impaired higher brain function, such as impaired judgment, speech difficulties, aggression, angry outbursts, impaired visuospatial abilities (ability to perceive time and manipulate objects in space), impaired impulse control, and disinhibition. Visuospatial disturbances often interfere with the ability to drive or draw a geometric figure on the MMSE. Deterioration of these brain regions is associated with behavioral and psychiatric disturbances in the patient with AD. Neuroanatomic studies, such as magnetic resonance spectroscopy, and assessment tools used to measure cognitive decline such as the MMSE, reveal degenerative processes and global cognitive deficits in patients with AD.[44] Because of the degenerative and progressive course of AD, behavioral and psychiatric disturbances are likely to contribute to the family or caregivers seeking evaluation and treatment in vast clinical settings.

### Acute Management of Behavioral and Psychiatric Symptoms

Presently there is no cure for AD, so treatment focus is on preserving cognitive functioning, reducing behavioral problems, and delaying dementia progression while maximizing quality of life.[45] Cholinesterase inhibitors, including donepezil, rivastigmine, and galantamine, are first-line AD medications that can help improve memory, thinking, language, and judgment. Only donepezil is approved for all stages of AD, whereas rivastigmine and galantamine are limited to mild or moderate AD. The noncompetitive N-methyl-D-aspartate–receptor antagonist memantine is indicated in moderate to severe AD, targeting glutamate activity to slow memory loss and improve attention.[45,46] Acute management begins with establishing rapport with the patient, family members, and caregivers; using data to determine an accurate diagnosis; and initiating appropriate interventions.

### Assessment and Diagnosis

Approaching the patient and family members in a concerned, unhurried, and empathetic manner is key to establishing rapport and facilitating the data-gathering process. In addition, using active listening skills, offering reassurance, and attending to unmet needs offer comfort and safety.

The MMSE offers relevant data about cognitive function. Recent and remote memory difficulties are hallmark symptoms of AD and often indicate an inability to learn new information or retrieve stored information. In addition to the questions mentioned with assessing the patient with delirium, nurses need to ask caregivers concerning the duration of symptoms, if the patient has been getting lost, current driving patterns, traffic accidents, and ability to maintain self-care. Similarly to assessing the patient with delirium, a patient presenting with memory and other cognitive deficits requires a comprehensive physical and psychosocial assessment. Memory deficits often signal alterations in mental functioning and are the initial indication of dementia. When it is determined that the patient has dementia, interventions to reduce psychosis and aggression and other behavioral disturbances must be initiated to promote comfort and safety in staff, the patient, and caregivers.

### Interventions

Patients with AD exhibit an array of symptoms, including psychosis, agitation, and verbal aggression. Major treatment goals must include abating delusions, hallucinations, and suspiciousness and concurrent behavioral disturbances. Significant behavioral disturbances are screaming, agitation, restlessness, cursing, combativeness, and violence. Treating AD requires an interdisciplinary and holistic approach that focuses on safety and maintenance of the patient's global psychosocial, nutritional, physical, and functional needs and integrity. The treatment approach also must integrate the needs of caregivers by reducing their distress through reassurance, health education, and appropriate community referrals. These patient-centered approaches must combine psychosocial, environmental, health education, and pharmacologic interventions that ultimately facilitate a sense of dignity, promote safety, and promote comfort.

A wide range of underlying causative triggers can manifest as behavioral disruptions, such as environmental changes, hunger, fecal impaction, medication side effects, depression, infection, covert fall, urinary tract infection pain, loneliness, or exacerbation of underlying illness.[45,47,48] Environmental interventions involve using calendars, pictures, and clocks as environmental cues and soothing approaches using music and pet therapy and other measures to reduce frustration and agitation and to enhance comfort and relaxation. Environmental interventions also include assessing the family members' ability to care for the patient and their level of distress.

Managing psychotic and behavioral disturbances must be governed by the severity of symptoms and level of patient distress or dangerousness. When the situation is deemed dangerous because of combativeness, hallucinations, or paranoia, pharmacologic and other interventions must be considered to ensure safety. Target treatment symptoms include hallucinations, delusions, agitation, verbal abuse, and physical aggression—the most distressing characteristics of AD. Unresolved or inadequate management of psychotic and behavioral symptoms of dementia contributes to caregiver burnout, eroded quality of life, and institutional placement. Additional safety measures have been referenced previously.

Antipsychotics were once considered a primary pharmacotherapy for psychotic and behavioral disturbances in dementia, with SGA considered especially promising due to efficacy treating psychosis and combativeness without the conventional antipsychotic extrapyramidal effects. The US Food and Drug Administration has since declared that neither conventional nor atypical antipsychotics are indicated for the treatment of dementia-related psychosis due to their increased risks of stoke and death. However, the clinical consequences of unmanaged psychotic and behavioral disturbances in dementia are also dangerous, and off-label antipsychotic use in dementia treatment persists. Risks may be tempered by treating the underlying causative behaviors triggers, ensuring appropriate biopsychosocial interventions, applying previously effective strategies, consultation with family/caregivers and patient (when possible), consideration of medication impact on quality of life and safety, slow titration until therapeutic response or emergence of side effects, and reassessment for tolerability and risks/benefits for continued use.[45,49,50]

Health education is an integral part of caring for the patient with AD because the patient's dependency needs and disruptive behaviors increase the risk of elder abuse and caregiver burden. Health education needs to center on the course of AD, including mild to severe symptoms, available treatment options and related behavioral management, and respite care. If the early symptoms exist, the patient and family members must deal with legal issues and future symptoms and options and identify emergent situations and when to seek medical attention. Family members are often in denial because of the stigma attached to AD and other behavioral problems and need reassurance. They must also deal with personal issues that threaten the patient's dignity and potential caregiver's burden. Social and community referrals also must be provided to assist caregivers in dealing with their own stressors inherent in caring for the patient with AD.[51]

### Evaluation

Evaluating treatment outcomes in the management of behavioral and psychotic disturbances in patients with AD is based on the patient's response to treatment and safe resolution of acute symptoms. Nurses must assess the patient response to treatment continuously and reassure family members about their loved one's condition.

### SUMMARY

As the population ages, nurses in various clinical settings must identify high-risk groups that are vulnerable to delirium and dementia. They also must be able to provide psychosocial and pharmacologic interventions that promote comfort and safety for the patient and their families experiencing these distressful medical conditions. Efforts to facilitate healthy resolution and restore the patient and caregivers to an optimal level of function must be priorities.

### REFERENCES

1. Administration on Aging, Administration for Community Living, U.S. Department of Health and Human Services. A profile of older Americans: 2014. 2014. Available at: http://www.aoa.acl.gov/Aging_Statistics/Profile/2014/docs/2014-Profile. pdf. Accessed November 10, 2015.
2. Centers for Disease Control and Prevention. Older persons' health. Atlanta (GA): FastStats; 2015. Available at: http://www.cdc.gov/nchs/fastats/older-american-health.htm.
3. De Lange E, Verhaak PFM, van der Meer K. Prevalence, presentation and prognosis of delirium in older people in the population, at home and in long term care: a review. Int J Geriatr Psychiatry 2013;28(2):127–34.
4. Wass S, Webster PJ, Nair BR. Delirium in the elderly: a review. Oman Med J 2008; 23(3):150–7. Available at: http://www.ncbi.nlm.nih.gov/pmc/articles/PMC3282320/.
5. Gower LEJ, Gatewood MO, Kang CS. Emergency department management of delirium in the elderly. West J Emerg Med 2012;13(2):197–201.
6. Salluh J, Soares M, Teles J, et al. Delirium epidemiology in critical care (DECCA): an international study. Crit Care 2010;14(6):R210.

7. Inouye SK, Robinson T, Blaum C, et al. Postoperative delirium in older adults: best practice statement from the American Geriatrics Society. J Am Coll Surg 2015; 220(2):136–48.

8. Miller MO. Evaluation and management of delirium in hospitalized older patients. Am Fam Physician 2008;78(11):1265–70. Available at: http://www.aafp.org/afp/2008/1201/p1265.html#afp20081201p1265-b4.

9. Siddiqi N, House AO, Holmes JD. Occurrence and outcome of delirium in medical in-patients: a systematic literature review. Age Ageing 2006;35(4):350–64.

10. Harrington CJ, Vardi K. Delirium: presentation, epidemiology, and diagnostic evaluation (part 1). R I Med J 2014;97(6):18–23. Available at: https://www.rimed.org/rimedicaljournal/2014/06/2014-06-18-psych-harrington.pdf.

11. American Psychiatric Association. Diagnostic and statistical manual of mental disorders: DSM-5. 5th edition. Arlington (VA): American Psychiatric Association; 2013.

12. Cole MG, Ciampi A, Belzile E, et al. Persistent delirium in older hospital patients: a systematic review of frequency and prognosis. Age Ageing 2009;38(1):19–26.

13. Vidal EO, Boas PJF, Valle AP, et al. Delirium in older adults. Br Med J 2013;346: f2031.

14. Toor R, Liptzin B, Fischel SV. Hospitalized, elderly, and delirious: what should you do for these patients? Curr Psychiatry 2013;12(8):10–8. Available at: http://www.currentpsychiatry.com/home/article/hospitalized-elderly-and-delirious-what-should-you-do-for-these-patients/718bf7443e66064acf1122610db75ef3.html.

15. Inouye SK, Van Dyck CH, Balkin CA, et al. Clarifying confusion: the confusion assessment method. A new method for detection of delirium. Ann Intern Med 1990;113(12):941–8.

16. Anderson P. New 3-minute delirium test. Medscape Nurses 2014. Available at: http://www.medscape.com/viewarticle/833600.

17. Marcantonio ER, Ngo LH, O'Connor M, et al. 3D-CAM: derivation and validation of a 3-minute diagnostic interview for CAM-Defined delirium: a cross-sectional diagnostic test study. Ann Intern Med 2014;161(8):554–61.

18. Boettger S, Breitbart W. Phenomenology of the subtypes of delirium: phenomenological differences between hyperactive and hypoactive delirium. Palliat Support Care 2011;9(2):129–35.

19. Lorenzl S, Füsgen I, Noachtar S. Acute confusional states in the elderly. Dtsch Arztebl Int 2012;109(21):391–400.

20. Yang FM, Marcantonio ER, Inouye SK, et al. Phenomenological subtypes of delirium in older persons: patterns, prevalence, and prognosis. Psychosomatics 2009;50(3):248–54.

21. Kiely DK, Jones RN, Bergmann MA, et al. Association between psychomotor activity delirium subtypes and mortality among newly admitted postacute facility patients. J Gerontol A Biol Sci Med Sci 2007;62(2):174–9.

22. King J, Gratrix A. Delirium in intensive care. Continuing Education in Anesthesia, Critical Care & Pain 2009;9(5):144–7. Available at: http://ceaccp.oxfordjournals.org/content/9/5/144.full.

23. Schwartz JR, Roth T. Neurophysiology of sleep and wakefulness: basic science and clinical implications. Curr Neuropharmacol 2008;6(4):367–78.

24. Mergenhagen KA, Arif S. Delirium in the elderly: medications, causes, and treatment. Lyndhurst (NJ): US Pharmacist; 2008. Available at: http://www.uspharmacist.com/continuing_education/ceviewtest/lessonid/105762/.

25. Luukkanen MJ, Uusvaara J, Laurila JV, et al. Anticholinergic drugs and their effects on delirium and mortality in the elderly. Demen Geriatr Cogn Dis Extra 2011;1(1):43–50.

26. Chan PKY. Clarifying the confusion about confusion: current practices in managing geriatric delirium. Br Columbia Med J 2011;53(8):409–15. Available at: http://www.bcmj.org/sites/default/files/BCMJ_53_Vol8_delirium.pdf.

27. Inouye SK, Charpentier PA. Precipitating factors for delirium in hospitalized elderly persons. J Am Med Assoc 1996;275(11):852–7.

28. Zafirau B. Troubleshooting delirium in elderly inpatients. Norwalk (CT): Psychiatry Times; 2006. Available at: http://www.psychiatrictimes.com/articles/troubleshooting-delirium-elderly-inpatients.

29. Andrew MK, Freter SH, Rockwood K. Incomplete functional recovery after delirium in elderly people: a prospective cohort study. BMC Geriatr 2005;5:5.

30. Folstein MF, Folstein SE, McHugh PR. "Mini-mental state". A practical method for grading the cognitive state of patients for the clinician. J Psychiatr Res 1975; 12(3):189–98.

31. Vardi K, Harrington CJ. Delirium: treatment and prevention (part 2). R I Med J 2014;97(6):24–8. Available at: https://www.rimed.org/rimedicaljournal/2014/06/2014-06-24-psych-vardi.pdf.

32. Kalisvaart KJ, De Jonghe JFM, Bogaards MJ, et al. Haloperidol prophylaxis for elderly hip-surgery patients at risk for delirium: a randomized placebo-controlled study. J Am Geriatr Soc 2005;53(10):1658–66.

33. Teslyar P, Stock VM, Wilk CM, et al. Prophylaxis with antipsychotic medication reduces the risk of post-operative delirium in elderly patients: a meta-analysis. Psychosomatics 2013;54(2):124–31.

34. Maneeton B, Maneeton N, Srisurapanont M, et al. Quetiapine versus haloperidol in the treatment of delirium: A double-blind, randomized, controlled trial. Drug Des Devel Ther 2013;2013(7):657–67.

35. Markowitz JD, Narasimhan M. Delirium and antipsychotics: a systematic review of epidemiology and somatic treatment options. Psychiatry (Edgmont) 2008;5(10): 29–36. Available at: http://www.ncbi.nlm.nih.gov/pmc/articles/PMC2695757/.

36. Centers for Disease Control and Prevention. Alzheimer's disease. Atlanta (GA): Older Persons' Health; 2015. Available at: http://www.cdc.gov/aging/aginginfo/alzheimers.htm.

37. Corrada MM, Brookmeyer R, Paganini-Hill A, et al. Dementia incidence continues to increase with age in the oldest old: the 90+ study. Ann Neurol 2010;67(1): 114–21.

38. Asaad G. Hallucinations in clinical psychiatry: a guide for mental health professionals (Brunner/Mazel clinical psychiatry series). 1st edition. New York: Brunner/Mazel; 1990.

39. Steinberg M, Lyketsos CG. Atypical antipsychotic use in patients with dementia: managing safety concerns. Am J Psychiatry 2012;169(9):900–6.

40. Drouillard N, Mithani A, Chan PKY. Therapeutic approaches in the management of behavioral and psychological symptoms of dementia in the elderly. Br Columbia Med J 2013;55(2):90–5. Available at: http://www.bcmj.org/articles/therapeutic-approaches-management-behavioral-and-psychological-symptoms-dementia-elderly.

41. Sachdev PS, Blacker D, Blazer DG, et al. Classifying neurocognitive disorders: the DSM-5 approach. Nat Rev Neurol 2014;10:634–42.

42. Budson AE, Solomon PR. Memory loss: a practical guide for clinicians (expert consult—online). 2nd edition. New York: Saunders Title; 2014.

43. Stahl SM, Muntner N. Stahl's essential psychopharmacology: neuroscientific basis and practical applications. 4th edition. Cambridge (United Kingdom): Cambridge University Press; 2013.
44. Sheehan B. Assessment scales in dementia. Ther Adv Neurol Disord 2012;5(6): 349–58.
45. Sadowsky CH, Galvin JE. Guidelines for the management of cognitive and behavioral problems in dementia. J Am Board Fam Med 2012;25(3):350–66.
46. Davis JR. Alzheimer's disease: managing unique pharmacotherapy needs | page 1. Pharmacy Times 2015. Available at: http://www.pharmacytimes.com/publications/ health-system-edition/2015/january2015/alzheimers-disease-managing-unique- pharmacotherapy-needs/P-1.
47. Corbett A, Husebo BS, Achterberg WP, et al. The importance of pain management in older people with dementia. Br Med Bull 2014;111(1):139–48.
48. Sekerak RJ, Stewart JT. Black-box. Current Psychiatry 2014;22(12). Available at: http://www.annalsoflongtermcare.com/article/caring-patient-end-stage-dementia.
49. Steinberg M, Shao H, Zandi P, et al. Point and 5-year period prevalence of neuropsychiatric symptoms in dementia: the Cache County Study. Int J Geriatr Psychiatry 2008;23(2):170–7.
50. Meeks TW, Jeste DV. Antipsychotics in dementia: beyond 'black box' warnings. Curr Psychiatry 2008;7(6):50–65. Available at: http://www.currentpsychiatry. com/view-pdf.html?file=fileadmin/cp_archive/pdf/0706/0706CP_Article3.
51. Brodaty H, Donkin M. Family caregivers of people with dementia. Dialogues Clin Neurosci 2009;11(2):217–28. Available at: http://www.ncbi.nlm.nih.gov/pmc/ articles/PMC3181916/.

# Suicide: Across the Life Span

Jeffery Ramirez, PhD, PMHNP

## KEYWORDS

- Suicide • Risk factors • Adolescents • Older adults • Psychiatric • disorders
- Safety plan • Risk assessment

## KEY POINTS

- Suicide is a preventable act.
- Nurses in all practice settings must be able to conduct suicide risk assessments.
- Most patients who commit suicide have a history of a psychiatric disorder.
- Safety planning is an important aspect of nursing care for patients at risk for suicide.

## INTRODUCTION

Death by suicide continues to be a major public health problem. According to the Suicide Prevention Resource Center, suicide rates in the United States increased from 10.49 per 100,000 to 13.02 between the years of 2000 and 2013.[1] According to the Centers for Disease Control and Prevention (CDC), 41,149 suicide deaths occurred in 2013.[2] Furthermore, the American Foundation for Suicide Prevention reports the cost of treating nonfatal injuries due to self-harm is estimated at $2 billion annually. The indirect cost for lost wages and productivity is another $4.3 billion.[3] The rates of death by suicide continue to increase; at the same time there is decreasing rates of death by heart disease, cancer, and human immunodeficiency virus/AIDS.[4]

Professional nurses encounter patients at risk for suicide in all settings. These settings include community mental health, inpatient mental health, emergency units, and medical surgical units. All nurses must have the skill and competency to assess and intervene with patients experiencing suicidal thoughts and behaviors.

This article explores the explanations and descriptions of the cause of suicide from a neurobiological and psychological perspective, risk, and protective factors among high-risk groups, including youths and older adults. The article concludes with the responsibilities of nurses in the prevention, assessment, and treatment of people at risk for suicide.

Disclosure: None.
This article is an update of an article previously published in Nursing Clinics of North America, Volume 38, Issue 1, March 2003.
Department of Nursing and Human Physiology, Gonzaga University, 502 E. Boone Avenue, Spokane, WA 99258, USA
E-mail address: Ramirez@gonzaga.edu

## NEUROBIOLOGICAL AND PSYCHOLOGICAL THEORIES OF SUICIDE

Studies of suicide examine both neurobiological and psychological aspects. Neurobiological theories describe structural brain, genetic, and neurotransmitter changes. In contrast, psychological theories attempt to explain and describe the mental status of the person contemplating suicide by examining and analyzing their thoughts and behaviors. However, psychological and psychosocial aspects influence neurobiological changes in both the developing and adult brain.

## NEUROBIOLOGY OF SUICIDE

More than 90% of people dying by suicide have a major psychiatric disorder, primarily a mood disorder, such as depression.[5] In addition to a psychiatric disorder, other life stressors, such as traumatic events, influence changes in the brain and, therefore, have an impact on neurodegeneration and neuroplasticity.[5]

## CHANGES IN THE BRAIN AND NEUROTRANSMITTER SYSTEMS

The prefrontal cortex (PFC) is responsible for judgment and insight. People who have completed suicide had the ability to develop a well-thought-out plan, leave notes, generate a will, and notify friends and family. These actions indicate an intact, functioning PFC. The orbital prefrontal cortex (OPC) plays a key role in cognitive processing and decision-making and regulates emotions and the reward system. An impaired OPC reduces the ability to make and use serotonin. Serotonin is a critical neurotransmitter for regulating mood and impulse control, which provides an explanation of impulsive acts of suicide.[6,7] Autopsies indicate that the neurons in the dorsal raphe nucleus contain an enzyme that synthesizes serotonin, leading scientists to think the brain is trying to produce more serotonin. The dorsal raphe nucleus is the area of the brain for production of serotonin. People who completed suicide send less-than-normal amounts of serotonin to the OPC.[6,7]

Norepinephrine regulates the stress response, anxiety, and mood. There is increasing concentration of norepinephrine and alpha-adrenergic receptors, indicating the brain is attempting to produce more norepinephrine at the time of suicide. People who completed suicide have fewer norepinephrine transporters.[7,8]

## PSYCHOLOGICAL THEORIES OF SUICIDE

There are many theories attempting to explain and describe the psychache of the suicidal mine. *Psychache* is a term that was coined and defined by Shneidman[9] as unbearable psychological pain. In respect to this article, it refers to painful experiences that increase the risk of suicide. Researchers devoting their careers to the study of suicide are referred to as suicidologists. Most suicidologists conclude people dying by suicide experience an intense and inescapable sense of despair in regard to the subjective inability to tolerate internal experiences and responds to external circumstances.[10,11] People contemplating suicide want to live, but they see no option other than death. People thinking of suicide experience ambivalence up to the point of a suicide act. Suicidal ambivalence is the desire to live competing with the urge to die. Shneidman,[9] founder of modern suicidology, stated that out of all deaths we experience in our lives, suicide is the one we hate the most. He also states suicide is a permanent solution to a temporary problem. As nurses, we observe outsiders; but we need to remember the intense pain a person is experiencing blocks their ability to see any options to the situation except to escape through death.

## PSYCHOLOGICAL INFLUENCES

Risk factors are characteristics that increase the likelihood of suicidal behavior; however, they are not predictors or causes of suicide for any given individual. It is important to understand the distinction between a risk factor and risk predictors. Risk factors are characteristics that have been derived from researching a large sample of people who have completed suicide. Some examples of these characteristics include age, gender, and history. For example, people between 45 and 64 years of age had the highest rates; people 85 years and older had the second highest rates; men complete suicide at higher rates than women; people with a history of family members completing suicide are at higher risk than people without; whites have the highest rates, and American Indians and Alaska Natives have the second highest. The number one method of killing one self is with a firearm.[1] Risk predictors are characteristics of a person indicating the likelihood of suicide.[12] A person's risk for suicide will increase as personal risk factors accumulate; therefore, all risks warrant further scrutiny and assessment by the nurse.

Some psychological risk factors to consider are mood disorders, such as depression or bipolar; thought disorders, including schizophrenia, schizoaffective, or psychosis; substance abuse disorders; anxiety disorders; trauma- and stress-related disorders; and personality disorders, especially cluster B (antisocial, borderline, histrionic, or narcissistic). A person's risk increases if there is a presence of more than one disorder exacerbating psychiatric symptoms.[12]

## PSYCHOSOCIAL INFLUENCES

Stressful life events occur at different times in everybody's life. Some people are more vulnerable to stress leading to self-destructive behaviors and suicidal thoughts. Specific psychosocial stressors include loss, such as relationships, social, identity, status, work, or financial; family conflicts; legal issues, such as arrests or possibility of jail or prison sentence; lesbian, gay, bisexual, or transgender life style; failure in school; poor performance at a job; interpersonal conflict; self-hate; despair; low self-esteem; or feelings of hopelessness and helplessness.[12]

## ASSESSING PROTECTIVE FACTORS

Protective factors can be either internal or external strengths. Internal strengths include those interpersonal adaptive skills the person has used throughout life. External proactive factors are the patient's support systems and relationships. External protective factors include family, friends, and occupational security.[13] Protective factors shift suicidal ambivalence toward living and reduce the risk of suicide (**Box 1**).

## HIGH-RISK POPULATIONS
### Older Adults

The CDC reports people older than 85 years have the second highest rates of completed suicide among all age groups.[2] When an older adult attempts suicide, their risk of survival is diminished compared with their younger counterparts.

In 2012 the CDC reported the life expectancy is 78.8 years old.[2] People are living longer and, therefore, treatment and care needs increase. Not only are older adults challenged with chronic health conditions but they are also facing life changes, including loss of independence, spouses, friends, work, and social interactions. These interpersonal issues often lead to insomnia, depression, and anxiety.

---

**Box 1**
**Examples of protective factors**

- Thinks life has meaning or purpose
- Hopefulness and futuristic thinking
- Life has satisfaction
- Positive coping skills, conflict resolution, and nonviolent management of disputes
- Support systems, such as family, friends, and pets
- Spirituality or religious beliefs
- Sobriety
- Positive view of self
- Problem solving skills
- Lacks access to method of suicide

---

### Psychosocial factors

Various psychosocial issues have been mentioned previously. However, there are additional psychosocial risks nurses need to consider when working with an older adult at risk for suicide. As people age they are at risk of becoming more isolated and lack social connectedness. This circumstance leads to the beliefs of being a burden to others and thought patterns that others are better off if they were dead.[14] Additional reasons for late-life suicide attempts are[14,15] as follows:

- Somatic problems and pain
- Functioning and autonomy
- Social problems (belongingness or family conflict)
- Psychological problems
- Lack of meaning in life
- Stress
- Depression
- Hopelessness

As with all age groups, the risk factors need to be balanced with protective factors. As people age, they need to find meaning in life. A study by Heisel and Flett[15] (2015) found that elderly people had greater meaning in life with the following:

- Sense of well-being
- Sense of coherence
- Self-transcendence
- Resiliency
- Optimism
- Perceived social support

## TREATMENT CONSIDERATIONS
### Older Adults

The growing number of older adults in the United States and the high rates of suicide make suicide assessment a critical competency for nurses. The goal of caring for this population is preventing suicide. Screening tools for suicide, depression, and substance use should be made available to nurses because they are often the first health care professionals encountering patients.[16]

Late-life depression is common among the elderly with rates as high as 30% of all adults 65 years and older.[17] Additionally, older adults experience issues with insomnia, anxiety, and substance use. Symptoms of depression include decreased energy, sleep disturbance, weight changes, loss of interest, guilt, poor concentration, and thoughts of suicide. Treatment of depression includes psychoeducation, psychotherapy, and antidepressant medications.

Psychoeducation focuses on teaching coping strategies, assistance in finding social activities, and providing community resources. Another focus of psychoeducation is meeting with the family and provide education on suicide prevention strategies including recognizing warning signs and removing any lethal means, especially firearms.

Psychotherapy is used to treat both depression and anxiety. Cognitive-behavioral therapy (CBT) has been widely studies and has robust evidence as an effective treatment.[17] CBT is effective with older adults because it is time limited and helps recognize thought distortions and negative patterns. Once these thought patters are recognized, behavioral interventions are used to help individuals change, adapt, and develop new ways of viewing their life.[17]

Antidepressants have been safely used for older adults. Selective serotonin reuptake inhibitors are the preferred class of medications used in the elderly. These medications have a lower risk for adverse reactions than the tricyclic antidepressants and carry a lower risk of death if taken in an overdose. Older adults need assessing for polypharmacy and drug-drug interactions. Additionally, education regarding the correct administration of medications, frequency, and duration is necessary for patient safety.

### Youth

As previously mention, a strong relationship between depression and suicide has been established. In 2013, 2.6 million youths had major depression; 33.2% of these youths used illicit drugs.[18] The CDC estimates 4% of all suicide attempts are made by adolescents between 10 and 18 years of age.[2] Youths dying by suicide are the third leading cause of death among persons aged 10 to 14 years.[1] As with adults, boys complete suicide more often than girls, with some estimates as high as a 5 to 1 rations.[1] More than 3 million youths sought out mental health treatment of emotional and behavioral issues, and the most common reason for seeking treatment is for depressed moods.[2]

These data bring both good and bad news. Starting with the bad news, once a youth carries out the act of suicide and dies, there is no opportunity for treatment interventions. The good news is youths are seeking early treatment and providing early interventions improving outcomes. However, there are psychological and psychosocial factors to consider when caring for this population.

### Psychological considerations

Childhood is our most formative years for both physiologic and psychological growth. Neuroscience established that neuroplasticity allows the brain to change and adapt. Adolescents with depression have decreased volumes of prefrontal cortex, hippocampus, and amygdala.[19] The implications for these structural changes are poor decision-making, impulsivity, and poor emotional regulations. Furthermore, the right superior temporal gyrus is found to be smaller among adolescents with depression and a history of suicide attempts. The temporal gyrus plays a key role in attention, emotions, and spatial perceptions.[19] These changes in the brain have significant implications on the ability for youths to cope with the psychosocial demands in today's environment.

### Psychosocial considerations

A significant psychosocial issue causing harm to children and adolescents is in the form of bullying. There are multiple definitions; but bullying for the purpose of this discussion has 3 components to the definition by Liu and Grave[20] (2011): "(1) the bully's intention to cause harm to the victim, (2) the cause of harm being the perceived imbalance of power between the bully and the victim, and (3) the repetition of bullying behavior over time."[20]

One form of bullying receiving attention is cyberbullying. This form of bullying is through social media, such as Facebook, e-mails, chat rooms, Snapchat, Instagram, and texting, using computers, smartphones, iPads, and tablets. Bullying occurs when a bully posts rumors about the victim, sending obscene pictures, such as nude photographs of the victim, or sexual harassment. The goal of the bully is to cause harm to others through exclusion, harassment, threats, humiliation, and embarrassment. There is a direct correlation between cyberbullying and suicide risk. Studies concluded cyberbullying increases suicidal thoughts, which is a precursor to suicide.[21–23]

Other forms of bullying, such as verbal, physical, and sexual harassment, have the same consequences as cyberbullying. Adolescents present with unexplained psychosomatic symptoms, enuresis, sleep disturbances, decreased self-esteem, anxiety, and depression.[24]

### Sexual Minorities

Sexual minorities are at risk for suicide. It is established that lesbian, gay, bisexual, transgender, queer, and/or questioning adolescents struggle with being included in a peer group leading to increasing thoughts of suicide.[25]

## TREATMENT CONSIDERATIONS

The developmental phase the child or adolescent is in drives the treatment strategies. Treatment interventions have to build on the development strengths and competencies the child or adolescent have mastered. Additionally, psychosocial issues, such as bullying, sexual abuse, physical abuse, or depression, disrupt youths' emotional development; therefore, behaviors seem immature for their chronologic age.[26]

Treatment needs to involve the family as long as the family is not part of any abuse issues. Along with the social services that are needed, other treatment interventions include psychoeducation, medications, and psychotherapy. However, it is important to point out the risks of using antidepressants.

The Food and Drug Administration has a black box warning on all packages of antidepressants. The purpose of the warnings is to ensure providers, patients, and parents are aware of the risk. Children or adolescents need additional monitoring for any adverse side effects, especially increased suicidal thoughts. It is recommended that patients are monitored weekly for the first month, every other week for the next 4 weeks, and then 12 weeks after the initiation of therapy.[27]

## NURSING IMPLICATIONS AND TREATMENT
### Nurse Patient Relationship

Hildegard Peplau developed the interpersonal relations nursing theory. Peplau asserts that the relationship between the nurse and patients is the crux of psychiatric nursing. Peplau stated: "It seems to me that interpersonal relations is the core of nursing. Basically, nursing practice always involves a relationship between at least two real people—the nurse and the patient."[28] It is the therapeutic use of self that the nurse applies when relating to suicidal patients.

The interpersonal relations theory concerns itself with the elements in nursing that involve the nurse, patients, and what goes on between them.[29] This dynamic interaction involves the human experiences of both the nurse and patients. These human experiences cause actions and interactions of the thoughts, feelings, and behaviors from both the nurse and patients.

Building a therapeutic relationship, which is sometimes referred to as a therapeutic alliance, is critical to working with suicidal patients. Key concepts to understand building a therapeutic relationship[30] include the following:

- Trust: It depends on the feeling of being understood and accepted as a person.
- Respect: Patients are not judged on the behavior or what they report to the nurse.
- Understanding: The nurse is able to convey his or her understanding of the patients' emotional pain and anguish.
- Responsibility: Patients have the ability to recognize and accept responsibility for problem solving and changing their behaviors rather

Nurses working with suicidal patients must be self-aware of their own views and reactions to the idea of suicide. For example, nurses should ask themselves the following:

- Have I had a family member die by suicide? How does this affect me in my work?
- Have I had a friend or colleague die of suicide? How have I processed this?
- Is it wrong to take your own life? How did I come to this conclusion?

The practice of nursing requires self-reflection and self-awareness of one's own reactions when working with a person contemplating suicide. Managing one's reactions to suicide is an essential competency for building a therapeutic relationship.

Some nurses may be reluctant to discuss suicide because they fear it will give patients the idea. Our understanding is a person thinking of suicide thought of it long before he or she sought treatment. Asking directly about suicidal intent lowers anxiety and decreases suicidal risk.

### Therapeutic Communication Techniques

Shea[12] (2011) developed techniques to help uncover complex secrets. Shea described 6 concepts for building a relationship with someone thinking about suicide and provided these examples:

- Behavioral incident: This technique includes any question in which the nurse asks about concrete behavioral facts or trains of thought. This strategy uncovers secrets a person tries to conceal because of shame and humiliating content, such as sexual or physical abuse.
- Shame attenuation: This technique assists the nurse inquiring about topics patients find embarrassing or shaming and too difficult to discuss.
- Gentle assumption: This technique is similar to shame attenuation; it increases the likelihood that patients become more open to discussing sensitive topics and allow the nurse to uncover secretes.
- Symptom amplification: This technique is useful if the nurse thinks patients are minimizing symptoms. This line of questioning is useful to obtain more accurate information, allowing the nurse to probe for very specific details.
- Normalization: Nurses help patients relax and decrease their anxiety using normalization. This technique gives patients validation that others in similar situations experience the same responses.[12]

## Assessment of Suicidal Patients

Listening skills are essential to nursing care. Communication strategies seek out evidence of overwhelming emotional pain, hurt, and anguish through verbal and nonverbal language. It is thought that every case of suicide stems from excessive and intense emotional pain. In addition, assessing for lethality is critical. Lethality is defined as the real danger to life associated with a suicide method or plan. The nurse must inquire about the plan and method. The level of lethality parallels suicide risk. Patients' risk increases especially if there is a detailed plan and access to a high method of lethality, such as a firearm (**Box 2**).

Some patients demonstrate behavior and cognitive clues. Patients may have difficulty sleeping or vegetative symptoms. Often they have difficulty problem solving and display poor judgment. Patients with tunnel vision and poor problem-solving skills are at extremely high risk. Patients experiencing hallucinations with themes of guilt, worthlessness, or the need to die pose a high risk. Some questions to assess for behavioral or cognitive clues are as follows:

- Have there been changes in your sleep pattern?
- What are the voices telling you to do?
- Is there anything troubling about your thoughts?

If a nurse is suspicious patients are at risk for suicide, an assessment of patients' affective state needs to be completed. A person's affect is defined as a person's emotional state or mood. If a person is showing increased signs of depression, then the nurse must assess further. Patients may have an increase in anxiety, irritability, self-hatred, shame, guilt, and hopelessness.

Sample questions are as follows:

- What do you think will happen in the future?
- Do you hurt or suffer so badly that you do not want to go on living?
- Is there anything you think you need to be punished for?
- Do you think a time will come when you will feel better?

## Assessing Suicide Risk

A thorough assessment of patients' history is critical to obtain accurate data. Any previous diagnosis or the presence of psychiatric disorders indicates neurobiological and psychological vulnerabilities to suicide. Key areas of assessing are as follows:

- Previous suicide attempts
- Family history of suicide or suicide attempts
- Self-injurious behaviors

---

**Box 2**
**Sample questions to use to assess for suicidal thoughts**

- Do you have current or past thoughts of suicide? If you are currently having thoughts, please describe them. What has stopped you from acting on these thoughts?

- Some people who are as upset as you sometimes have thoughts of suicide or wish they were dead. Are you feeling that way too?

- It seems that you are getting things in order. Are you thinking about suicide?

- What has been keeping you alive?

- Do you have access to firearms?

- Family history of a psychiatric disorder
- Family history of substance use disorder
- Impulsive or explosive reactions and behaviors[31,32]
- Childhood trauma, including being a trauma survivor of abuse, whether sexual, physical, or emotional; witnessing interpersonal violence; or growing up in a household with substance use or psychiatric disorder

Physical and sexual abuses between 16 and 25 years of age have correlated with suicide attempts and ideations. As many as 33% of women and 50% of men who attempted suicide experienced some form of abuse.[27]

Nurses must continuously assess patients at risk for suicide. This assessment includes completing and documenting a mental status examination and a suicide risk assessment. Other nursing interventions include the following:

- Treat patients with empathy and instill hope.
- Be aware of high-risk times, such as admission to an inpatient unit, change of shift, transfer to another unit, discharge, returning to court or other legal issues, and receiving disturbing news, such as loss of a loved one.
- Never leave patients alone.
- Initiate one-to-one observation when clinically indicated (staff must be trained to conduct this observation).
- Assess patients' ability to problem solve; in an acute state, patients will depend on the nursing staff. When patients are out of the acute state and problem solving, making hopeful statements, and looking toward the future, the nurse can teach effective coping strategies, including instructing patients on ways to manage intense internal emotions and self-sooth.
- Assist patients to recognize stressful situations that may trigger suicidal thoughts and then encourage patients to talk to someone about these thoughts.
- Help patients to focus on actions that empower and make a difference in their life. The nurse can encourage this by inviting simple decision-making and independence within the limits of patients' ability to promote recovery.
- Provide education to patients and families about psychiatric disorders, symptom management, and the stigma of having a psychiatric disorder.
- Provide a list of community resources at the time of discharge; teach patients how to access help, including 24-hour emergency hotline numbers, and what to do in a crisis.
- Teach patients and families the warning signs of suicide.
- Refer patients to the appropriate providers, particularly when working with outpatient settings, such as the emergency department or primary care.

### Suicide Contracts

Previous thoughts of using a suicide/safety contract, sometimes also called a no-suicide or no-harm contract, were intended to obtain an agreement with patients that they would not attempt suicide. These contracts, however, should not be viewed as an absolute safety measure for people being discharged or hospitalized because they are based on subjective data from patients and there is no objective evidence to demonstrate that patients will adhere to the agreement.

Suicide or safety contracts are not legal documents and cannot be used for the defense of a nurse if patients complete suicide. In fact, patients may be at greater risk with a suicide contract by giving the nurse a false sense of hope. A suicide contract must never be used with patients who are agitated, psychotic, impulsive, or under the influence of an intoxicating substance; they must also be avoided with people with borderline or passive-aggressive personalities. There is no evidence to support the use of suicide contracts.[12] However, development of a safety plan is a strength-based strategy for patient safety.

A suicide prevention strategy is using a safety plan. This strategy is different and should not be confused with a suicide contract because safety plans are considered best practice. Safety plans are developed with patients and their families. The first step is to remove the means patients plan to use. For example, if there are guns in the house, they need to be removed. The nurses need to assess the patients' understanding of the warning signs. Both the patients and families need to know the behaviors patients might exhibit, and patients need to recognize triggers. Once this has been established, then distracting activities need to be explored, such as listening to music, relaxing, or watching a movie. The final steps are to reach out to someone, such as a friend, family member, and ultimately a professional if needed.

## SUMMARY

Suicide can be prevented. The goal of all hospitals, communities, and all countries should be zero suicides. Nurses hold an important responsibility of preventing suicide because they spend the most time with patients out of all health care professionals.

Society is changing rapidly with the influences of technology and social media. The use of social media is increasing among younger populations and decreasing opportunities to develop interpersonal skills. The consequences are the inability to mange emotion and have sufficient coping skills during life changes.

Suicide risk assessment is a skill all nurses need to master in all work settings and extends beyond inpatient and outpatient psychiatric areas. For example, home health nurses doing visits are the first to recognize the risk of older adult patients and emergency department nurses are likely to encounter patients who attempted suicide. Furthermore, school nurses intervene with adolescents being bullied and can be the first to recognize the risk for suicide. Currently, there is no standard on how much time is devoted to suicide prevention and risk assessment. Therefore, the nursing profession must demand more time in nursing curriculums focused on suicide assessment and interventions.

## REFERENCES

1. Centers for Disease Control & Prevention (CDC). Injury prevention & control: data and statistics (WISQARS). Available at: http://www.cdc.gov/injury/wisqars/index.html. Accessed December 14, 2015.

2. Suicide facts at a glance 2015. Available at: www.cdc.gov/ViolencePrevention/pdf/Suicide-DataSheet-a.pdf; http://www.cdc.gov/injury/wisqars/index.html. Accessed December 14, 2015.

3. The American Foundation for Suicide Prevention facts and figures. Available at: http://www.afsp.org/understanding-suicide/facts-and-figures. Accessed November 27, 2015.

4. Fitzpatrick JJ. A national tragedy: increases in death by suicide, decreases in other major causes of death. Arch Psychiatr Nurs 2015;29:75.

5. Underwood MD, Arango V. Evidence for neurodegeneration and neuroplasticity as part of the neurobiology of suicide. Biol Psychiatry 2011;70:306–7.

6. Ding Y, Laueren N, Olie E, et al. Prefrontal cortex markers of suicidal vulnerability in mood disorders: a model based structural neuroimaging study with translational perspective. Transl Psychiatry 2015;5:1–8.

7. van Heeingen K, Mann JJ. The neurobiology of suicide. Lancet Psychiatry 2014; 1:63–72.
8. Oquendo MA, Sullivan GM, Sudol K, et al. Toward a biosignature for suicide. Am J Psychiatry 2014;171:1259–77.
9. Shneidman E. Autopsy of a suicide mind. New York: Oxford Press; 2004.
10. Orbach I. Taking an inside view: stories of pain. In: Michael K, Jobes DA, editors. Building a therapeutic alliance with the suicidal patient. Washington, DC: American Psychological Association; 2011. p. 111.
11. O'Connor RC, Nock MK. The psychology of suicidal behaviour. Lancet Psychiatry 2014;1:73–84.
12. Shea SC. The practical art of suicide assessment. Charleston (SC): Mental Health Presses; 2011.
13. Simon RI. Assessing protective factors against suicide: questioning assumptions. Psychiatr Times 2011;2011(28):35–41.
14. Van Orden KA, Wiktorsson S, Deberstein P, et al. Reasons for attempted suicide in latter life. J Geriatr Psychiatr 2015;23:536–44.
15. Heisel MJ, Flett GL. Does recognition of meaning in life confer resiliency to suicide ideation among community-residing older adults? A longitudinal investigation. J Geriatr Psychiatr 2015. http://dx.doi.org/10.1016/j.jagp.2015.02.007.
16. Erlangsen A, Nordentoft M, Conwell Y, et al. Key considerations for preventing suicide in older adults consensus opinions of an expert panel. Crisis 2011;32: 106–9. Hogrefe Publishing.
17. Steffens DC, Blazer DG, Thakur ME. The American psychiatric publishing textbook of geriatric psychiatry. 5th edition. Arlington (VA): American Psychiatric Publishing; 2015.
18. Substance Abuse and Mental health Services Administration. Results form the 2013 national survey on drug use and health: mental health findings, NSDUH Series H-49, HHS Publication No. (SMA). Rockville (MD): 2014. p. 14–4887.
19. Martin PC, Zimmer TJ, Pan LA. Magnetic resonance imaging markers of suicide attempts and suicide risk in adolescents. CNS Spectr 2015;20:355–8.
20. Liu J, Grave N. Childhood bullying: a review of constructs, concepts, and nursing implications. Public Health Nurs 2011;29(6):556–68.
21. Carpenter LM, Hubbard GB. Cyberbullying: implications for the psychiatric nurse practitioner. J Child Adolesc Psychiatr Nurs 2014;27:142–8.
22. Gini G, Espelage DL. Peer victimization, cyberbullying, and suicide risk in children and adolescents. JAMA 2014;32:545–6.
23. Hinduja S, Patchin JW. Bullying, cyberbullying, and suicide. Arch Suicide Res 2010;14:206–21.
24. Perron T. Looking at the factors associated with bullying and visits to the school nurse, in the United States. Br J Sch Nurs 2015;10:288–95.
25. Buchman-Schmitt JM, Chiruliza B, Chu C, et al. Suicidality in adolescent populations: a review of the extant literature through the lens of the interpersonal theory of suicide. Int J Behav Consult Ther 2014;9:26–34.
26. Estrine SA, Hettebach RT, Authur H, et al. Service delivery for vulnerable populations. New York: Springer Publishing; 2011.
27. Dilillio D, Mauri S, Mantegazz C, et al. Suicide in pediatrics: epidemiology, risk factors, warning signs, and the role of the pediatrician in detecting them. Ital J Pediatr 2015;41:49.
28. Fawcett J, DeSanto-Madeya S. Peplau's theory of interpersonal relations. In: Analysis and evaluation of contemporary nursing knowledge nursing models and theories. 3rd edition. Philadelphia: FA Davis; 2013. p. 382–98.

29. O'Toole AW, Welt SR. Interpersonal theory in nursing practices selected works of Hildegard E. Peplau. New York: Springer; 1989.
30. Michel K, Jobes D. Building a therapeutic alliance with the suicidal patient. Washington, DC: American Psychological Association; 2011.
31. Patel SC, Jakopac KA. Manual of psychiatric nursing skills. Sudbury (MA): Jones and Bartlett; 2012.
32. Dulcan M. Dulcan's textbook of child and adolescent psychiatry. Washington, DC: American Psychiatric Association Publishing; 2016.

# Psychosocial Recovery and Rehabilitation

Deborah Antai-Otong, MS, APRN, PMHCNS-BC, FAAN

## KEYWORDS

- Psychosocial rehabilitation • Cognitive remediation • Family involvement
- Symptomatic remission • Intensive case management • Self-efficacy
- Social cognition training • Supported employment

## KEY POINTS

- Discuss the history of psychosocial recovery and rehabilitation.
- Analyze the impact of self-efficacy and management of illness.
- Review the role of the nurse case manager as a member of the psychosocial rehabilitation team.
- Describe evidence-based pharmacologic and psychotherapeutic approaches used in the treatment of serious and chronic psychiatric and substance use conditions.
- Analyze major concepts of psychosocial rehabilitation and the recovery model.

Historically the term psychosocial rehabilitation was associated with individuals with serious mental illness and prominent functional impairment. Principal goals of these programs were symptom management and avoidance of rehospitalization. The goal of rehospitalization has been greatly abridged because of fewer inpatient hospital beds. Individuals who participated in these programs were not expected to fully recover nor were they given opportunities to fully integrate into their communities. Prevailing evidence indicates that individuals with severe psychiatric disorders, such as schizophrenia, bipolar disorder, and substance use disorders, share similar needs as those with chronic medical conditions (ie, diabetes, cardiovascular disorders). The issuance of the 2002 Executive Order of the President's New Freedom

The author has no financial interests to disclose.

This article is an update of an article previously published in Nursing Clinics of North America, Volume 38, Issue 1, March 2003.

All material appearing in this report is in the public domain and may be reproduced or copied without permission from SAMHSA. Citation of the source is appreciated. However, this publication may not be reproduced or distributed for a fee without the specific, written authorization of the Office of Communications, SAMHSA, HHS.

Department of Veterans Affairs, Veterans Integrated Service Networks-(VISN-17), 2301 E. Lamar Boulevard, Arlington, TX 76006, USA

E-mail address: Deborah.Antai-Otong@va.gov

Commission on Mental Health supported previous national guidance from the US Surgeon General that the provision of mental health services must be transformed from primarily symptoms management service and avoidance of hospitalization to one that uses evidence-based approaches that are person- and family-driven with emphasis on self-determined treatment choices and that center on a recovery model that instills hope, is strength-based, focuses on symptomatic remission, and builds resilience.[1–5] Recovery-oriented systems of care include the following concepts[5]:

- Hope and respect
- Complex and dynamic process
- Individualized and self-directed choices
- Comprehensive continuum of care
- Person-centered and responsive to person preferences, abilities, needs, and belief systems
- Community-integration
- Family or significant other involvement
- Culturally based
- Strength-based
- Integrated services
- Outcomes-driven and evidence-based

Psychosocial rehabilitation and mental health recovery is a dynamic and evidence-based model that provides a person-centered comprehensive, and seamless plan of care for patients with severe and persistent psychiatric illnesses. This model is closely linked to community integration that fosters a sense of belonging, provides integrated and comprehensive mental health services across a continuum of care, and facilitates family involvement and peer support and supported employment. Primary goals of this model include optimizing clinical and functional outcomes, sustaining recovery, and enriching quality of life.[1,5–7]

Major components of psychosocial recovery and rehabilitation include interventions that facilitate symptomatic remission, facilitate social cognition training, improve interpersonal relationships, and support and improve cognitive and functional performance. The goal of psychosocial rehabilitation has evolved from adherence to medication regimens and reduced hospitalization to helping the patient attain independence and sense of mastery and belonging, employment, meaningful interpersonal relationships, and an improved quality of life.[1–5] Ultimately, these goals facilitate the highest level of functioning in all spheres, self-efficacy, and well-being for patients with severe and persistent psychiatric conditions. By attaining these goals, patients with schizophrenia, bipolar disorder, and other severe and persistent psychiatric conditions can form supportive relationships, experience hope, and reduce symptoms and neurocognitive deficits that interfere with function and recovery. Predictably the success of these programs is enhanced by peer support and involvement of families and significant others.[7–10]

The concept of peer support has evolved the past few decades as a meaningful and productive approach based on helping patients with severe and persistent psychiatric illnesses.[7–10] Key tenets of this model are based on respect, personal accountability, mutual and shared experiences, and empathy. Peer support facilitates recovery through a reciprocal process of sharing experiences and tasks within structured psychosocial rehabilitation and mental health services. The ultimate goals of peer support and other recovery-based approaches are to sustain recovery as evidenced by optimal social functioning and integration into the community and improved quality of life. Achieving these goals requires integration by the interdisciplinary team model that involves the delivery of comprehensive, coordinated, person-centered, gender-based, and seamless services that are consumer-friendly and accessible to the patient, caregivers, and cultural and social context.[7–10]

Psychiatric nurses play pivotal roles in the implementation and efficacy of evidence-based psychosocial rehabilitation and are important members of interdisciplinary teams that provide holistic health care services ranging from symptom management to facilitating vocational rehabilitation. Psychiatric nurses, similar to other team members, patients, and caregivers, are also responsible for the planning and implementation of these services. This article focuses on psychosocial rehabilitation as an evidence-based practice model for the treatment of schizophrenia, bipolar disorders, and co-occurring psychiatric or substance-use disorders. The role of the psychiatric nurse in the planning and implementation of interdisciplinary interventions that instill hope and are strength-based, and that promote symptomatic remission, self-efficacy, assertive community treatment (ACT), psychoeducation, and vocational rehabilitation also is discussed.

## MAJOR COMPONENTS OF PSYCHOSOCIAL REHABILITATION AND MENTAL HEALTH RECOVERY

Studies underscore the significance of symptomatic remission, social skills building, and strengthening cognitive functioning to prepare patients for rehabilitation services and community integration.[1–5] Pharmacologic interventions are necessary to reduce or extinguish positive symptoms (ie, hallucination and delusions) and provide opportunities for the patient to develop and attain social and mental health rehabilitation and an optimal level of functioning and quality of life.[11,12] Psychiatric nurses are responsible for understanding the basis of medication, monitoring for desired responses and acute and chronic adverse drug reactions, and psychoeducation concerning psychiatric disorders and evidence-based treatment options. Regardless of the patient's condition, it is imperative for the nurse to identify symptoms and treatment options and to integrate the patient's strengths, abilities, preferences, and needs into person-centered treatment planning.

## SYMPTOMATIC REMISSION

The initial phase of psychosocial rehabilitation begins during the acute phase, at which time the primary goal is controlling and stabilizing positive symptoms of severe psychiatric disorders, often with pharmacologic interventions. Depending on the nature of the symptoms, various medications are used. The mainstay treatment of serious and chronic psychiatric disorders is pharmacotherapy and psychotherapeutic interventions.[11–15] Predictably the patient's presenting symptoms determine the exact medication. Patients with schizophrenia may enter treatment with acute psychosis. Efforts to assess the underlying cause of the acute symptoms must involve making a differential diagnosis. Nurses often are involved and gather crucial data, including assessing vital signs, drug toxicology screens, and chemistry profiles; performing a mental status examination; assessing danger to self and others; and obtaining an extensive substance abuse history that provides information about symptoms, duration, past treatment, and current medication.

After acute psychosis remits, atypical agents are preferred for maintenance treatment of psychotic disorders because of a reduced risk of producing permanent involuntary movement disorders (ie, tardive dyskinesia). During the past decade the Food and Drug Administration has approved a plethora of atypical antipsychotic medications that include quetiapine, asenapine, aripiprazole, lurasidone, brexpipra-zole (also used as adjunct treatment antidepressants), and cariprazine.[13,14] Atypical antipsychotic agents are preferred for maintenance treatment of psychotic disorders because of their reduced risk of producing permanent involuntary movement disor-ders (ie, tardive dyskinesia). Newer agents have additional advantages over typical agents because they target brain regions associated with negative symptoms of schizophrenia, such as mood, affect, cognitive disturbances, and facial expression related to underlying emotion states. Researchers assert that negative symptoms are associated with impaired cognitive and psychosocial functioning, poor quality of life, and negative treatment outcomes (See Courtney J. Givens: Adverse Drug Reactions Associated with Antipsychotic, Antidepressants, Mood Stabilizers, and Stimulants, in this issue and Lisa Jensen: Managing Acute Psychotic Disorders in an Emergency Department, in this issue concerning nursing implications for the man-agement of acute psychosis and side effects related to the use of typical and atypical side effects).[12,13,15] Short-term hospitalization is often required to stabilize medical and psychiatric symptoms or referral to a day hospital program or individual psycho-therapist to continue psychosocial recovery and rehabilitation.

Because of notable advantages of atypical antipsychotic agents, patients with serious and persistent psychiatric illnesses are more likely to reach an optimal level of function when this approach is integrated with psychotherapeutic interventions. Of particular importance to medication management is family and patient psychoedu-cation and social cognition training, such as cognitive remediation. This approach tar-gets negative symptoms related to cognitive and psychosocial deficits associated with schizophrenia and other severe and persistent psychiatric disorders. Re-searchers submit that integrating these components into psychosocial rehabilitation treatment planning help patients practice real life social, vocational, and interpersonal skills; enhance their quality of life; and sustain recovery.[11,12,14,15]

## SELF-EFFICACY AND MANAGEMENT OF ILLNESS

As patients transition from the acute symptom management stage, psychiatric nurses must monitor their response to treatment and provide opportunities for success. As the nurse administers or prescribes neuroleptic agents, it is imperative to educate the patient and significant others about schizophrenia or other serious mental disor-ders, reasons for medications, and potential side effects. This process facilitates insight into the patient's symptoms and illness and promotes self-efficacy as the pa-tient moves through the treatment continuum. Understandably, psychiatric rehabilita-tion evolves during the acute stages of a psychiatric disorder and continues throughout the life span. Mental health services must parallel stages of symptoms across the treatment continuum and meet the patient's holistic needs and foster competence and management of illness. Self-management of illness often requires structured interventions that promote self-efficacy, independence, employment, qual-ity interpersonal relationships, and a good quality of life. Self-efficacy and manage-ment of symptoms are crucial to moving from inpatient to community-based settings. Throughout the course of treatment, patient and family needs must be assessed thoroughly so that they can guide treatment planning and facilitate compe-tence in managing symptoms and responsibility for treatment outcomes. Dhillon and Dollieslager[16] delineated five core objectives of psychosocial rehabilitation as follows:

- Assess the patient's personal goals in life based on his or her strengths, prefer-ences, abilities, needs, including self-efficacy, autonomy, and quality of time with

friends and family, and how they can be facilitated by inpatient rehabilitation and symptomatic remission.
- Provide health education to the patient and significant others concerning the nature of the psychiatric illness and how medications and psychotherapeutic interventions may be useful in restoring self-control.
- Educate the patient about medication and treatment of adverse effects and the importance of self-monitoring and collaborating with the nurse or other health care provider concerning medication and its effect.
- Embrace the patient's culture and needs and collaborate with the family or other community-based resources.
- Engage the patient in decision making regarding appropriate discharge planning to facilitate community integration and plans for residential and other treatment needs.

## PSYCHOTHERAPEUTIC INTERVENTIONS
### Intensive Case Management

Traditionally, case management did not meet the needs of patients with schizophrenia or other serious and chronic psychiatric and substance-use disorders because patients were referred to a single case manager who functioned as a broker of services, rather than being assigned to an integrated community-based treatment team. Case management refers to the coordination, integration, and allocation of holistic care within a spectrum of resources. This concept has evolved over the years to overcome deficiencies in community-based mental health care and correct fragmented care and lack of continuity of care.[17] Despite earlier efforts to address these concerns the traditional case management model was unsuccessful in reducing hospitalization with little evidence of improving mental health social functioning, clinical outcome, or quality of life. This older model had high caseloads and used an individual versus a team approach to access patient resources, emphasizing community team outreach rather than referring the patient to other providers. This may have been related to the model's failure to reflect the relevance of cognitive and social skills necessary to follow up with appointments and get one's needs met. Combined, these factors placed the patient at risk of relapse and adverse clinical outcomes, including suicide and incarceration.

A contemporary approach to intensive case management is the ACT program.[17–20] With this approach, the patient is assigned to an interdisciplinary community team that includes a case manager, nurse, and other providers. ACT team members have lower caseloads than their predecessors. Care planning and interventions focus on a continuity of care model that includes coordination of various services and resources that feature outreach and affording in-home services. There is high staff-to-patient ratio that delivers services when and where needed by the patient, 24 hours a day, 7 days a week.[17–19]

Historically, the primary goal of intensive case management was the prevention of rehospitalization, but because of the shortage of inpatient beds this is no longer practicable. Reducing rehospitalization in high-risk patients through the provision of comprehensive integrated community services is cost-effective and a necessary component of this approach. Most researchers looking for cost-effective mental health services for individuals with serious and chronic psychiatric disorders have found that the ACT model program consistently shows reduced hospitalization and stability in the community.[17–19] The case manager role in the ACT program is especially suitable for the nurse because nurses in general have been health care brokers, providers of mental health care, and active members of the interdisciplinary team.

Ideally, as a case manager, the nurse within an interdisciplinary team oversees and integrates seamless, coordinated, and person-centered and shared decision-making treatment planning and facilitates patient access to appropriate community services.[18,19] An integral aspect of an intensive case management program is social skills training and vocational rehabilitation. Implementation of these components further strengthens rehabilitation, promotes recovery and a higher level of functioning, and improves quality of life.

### Social Cognition Training, Rehabilitation, and Recovery

Intensive case management programs, such as ACT, offer a wealth of opportunities to provide effective and individualized mental health services to patients with serious and chronic psychiatric disorders. Another aspect of integrated services using this model is social skills training. Psychiatric nurses involved in social skills training must do a comprehensive biopsychosocial assessment and determine the patient's mental and physical health, present and past coping skills, trauma history, quality of interpersonal relationships, strengths, preferences, abilities and needs, and readiness for training and rehabilitation. Psychiatric nurses also provide health education, health counseling, and medication management to ensure safety and facilitate recovery and optimal health. To determine the patient's readiness for social cognition training and rehabilitation, symptomatic management and cognition must be assessed.[11,21,22] Social cognition deficits, particularly negative symptoms (ie, perceptual disturbances), are widely accepted as contributing factors in functional and quality of life outcomes in patients with serious and chronic psychiatric disorders (ie, schizophrenia, bipolar disorders). These areas are also targets for social cognition training. As previously discussed, medications, specifically novel atypical or atypical antipsychotic medications, seem to be the mediator between social functioning and social cognition performance.[13,14,21,22]

Social cognition training refers to necessary competencies that allow for optimal social performance. Social cognition training uses learning theory principles to facilitate optimal social and community functioning, including activities of daily living, employment, leisure, and interpersonal relationships. The premise of this training is that it affords the patient opportunities to reach an optimal level of functioning and self-efficacy and community integration.

Bellack and Mueser[23] described two models of social skills training: basic and social problem solving. The basic model involves corrective learning, practiced through various means, including role playing. If the patient lacks assertive communication skills, the nurse can teach these skills and enhance them through role playing and constructive feedback. The social problem-solving model, such as cognitive remediation, focuses on improving information processing assumed to result in social skills deficits. Major foci for the social problem-solving model include requiring changes in medication and symptomatic remission, leisure, communication skills, and self-care. Each domain is taught in a module format with the goal of correcting receptive, processing, and transmitting skills deficits. Nursing interventions that promote these changes include providing examples of potential situations and asking the patient to think of possible solutions. When these solutions are presented, the nurse can offer feedback and options for improving communication and problem-solving skills. These solutions also may include medication side effects and possible ways to resolve them, including whether to call the provider concerning their effects. The premise underlying the cognitive remediation paradigm includes targeting cognitive deficits in attention, distorted self-evaluation; and planning goal-directed actions and helping the patient understand personal experiences associated with psychosis and emotional processes.[11,21,22] Nursing interventions involving this approach include establishing rapport and asking questions about upcoming situations, such as employment, conflict management, or need for medication changes. By offering these "real life" scenarios and teaching the patient basic interpersonal and problem-solving skills to resolve them, the nurse helps the patient understand personal experiences associated with psychosis and develop adaptive ways to resolve them, resulting in improved symptom-remission, confidence, self-efficacy, and recovery.

### Psychoeducation and Family Therapy

The global burden of serious psychiatric disorders, such as schizophrenia and bipolar disorder, is profound and often extends to the family, culture, and community. Efforts to strengthen family- and community-based resources are crucial to successful reintegration into the community and prevention of rehospitalization. The ACT program has been mentioned as one aspect of this process. Another aspect of the ACT program requires family or significant other involvement. Family involvement is generally acknowledged as a key factor in patient functional outcomes, recovery, and quality of life. Because of the intimate role that nurses play in mental health treatment planning, they must play key roles in identifying family, patient, cultural beliefs about causes and meaning of symptoms, and community stressors and strengths and collaborate with other members of the treatment team to support and empower family coping skills. Family stress often manifests as expressed emotion or an index of criticism, overinvolvement, and hostility. The expressed emotion and impaired family functioning research demonstrates that when levels of emotion or stress are reduced, so are psychotic relapses.[24,25]

Research consistently shows that the vulnerability-stress paradigm of schizophrenia suggests that patients with serious and chronic psychiatric and substance use disorders are likely to return to the hospital when community resources including family support are inadequate.[24,25] Because schizophrenia and other severe and persistent psychiatric and substance use disorders are costly and labor intensive, efforts to strengthen the family and community resources during these times are crucial to the mental health of the patient and community. Multifamily groups enable members to express their feelings and concerns about living with someone with a chronic mental disorder and promote self-management of illness. Nursing implications from this premise include assessing family stressors, perception of symptoms and disorders, coping and learning styles, and identifying family strengths, and providing health education that enables family members to understand their loved one's symptoms and ways to manage them and to facilitate health coping skills. Working with other team members and community agencies provides numerous opportunities for the patient and family to strengthen their coping skills and develop successful treatment recovery and functional outcomes. Psychiatric nurses must work with the patient and family to formulate and implement a person-centered comprehensive intervention program that eventually includes reducing dosages of antipsychotic medication, relying on novel medications to control symptoms and improve cognitive deficits, and implementing psychosocial interventions that integrate individualized needs of the patient and family.

There are many psychosocial family interventions, including those that begin on inpatient units and continue on an outpatient basis. One such program has been established for first-episode psychosis and has a 1-year, phase-specific, community-oriented treatment mode or specialized early interventions.[26,27] This approach advocates the importance and long-term benefits of early intervention in the treatment of first-episode psychosis. Researchers using this model submit that poor outcomes are linked to delayed treatment, lack of integration, and lack of medical and psychosocial interventions.[26–28] Support for this approach continues to demonstrate great promise because it provides treatment on a continuum that begins during the acute period and continues into the community.[26–28] Major goals of this model include bolstering the patient's activities of daily living skills, improving communication skills, and providing mutual support during the transitional phase of recovery from acute psychosis. This program is based on a structured 8-week model that reflects various themes, including self-identity, health education concerning the definition of psychosis, peer pressure and substance-related disorders, family and social interactions and medications, stigma, social skills and recovery, return to work or school, and warning signs of relapse. When patients complete this introductory phase, cognitive-oriented skills training is introduced and implemented over a 10-week period.

As with most models, family intervention is an integral part of this training; this particular model for first-episode psychosis is based on Anderson and colleague's[29] psychoeducation and management teaching model, modified to address the specific needs of younger first-episode patients. A period of engagement, initial crisis resolution, social support, and a series of psychoeducation workshops strengthen the patient and family's coping skills and assist them in managing various stressors associated with having a serious and chronic mental disorder. This psychoeducation model was designed for first-episode psychosis, but major components can be modified to meet the needs of most patients experiencing a serious and chronic mental illness. Psychiatric nurses play pivotal roles in working with the patient with serious mental disorders from the acute stage to the transition to family and community-based settings. Throughout the treatment process, patients must be empowered and encouraged to take responsibility for their recovery. Through self-efficacy activities, family involvement, and psychoeducation, the patient gains a sense of independence and confidence to seek and form quality interpersonal relationships, initially with the nurse and later through family interactions, peer support, and community integration. As these skills evolve, so too does confidence that propels the patient to participate in workshops and other community employment. Nurses must offer opportunities for the patient and family to identify and express concerns as consumers and promote a good quality of life.

### Supported Employment

Ultimately, psychosocial rehabilitation prepares the patient for supported employment.[18,19,30,31] Evaluations for supported employment are conducted by vocational rehabilitation and/or occupational specialists. Major advantages of these programs include helping the patient make person-centered choices based on their strengths, abilities, preference, and needs and shared-decision making, and acquire necessary skills to maintain competitive and gainful employment. These programs also offer incentives for patients with severe and chronic psychiatric and substance use disorders to increase their autonomy as recovery or rehabilitation progresses. In addition to benefiting the patient, supported employment adds to the workforce and community. Nurse case managers also provide prospects to participate in supportive psychotherapy and problem solving that assist the patient in daily problems and coping with his or her illness. Through structured or supervised workshops and work programs, patients gain a sense of self-worth and independence and develop interpersonal relationships that involve family members and peers. Research studies indicate that a major barrier to supported employment is access despite increasing use. It is imperative for nurses to stress the importance of self-management and deal with substance use disorders.

As the patient regains hope and moves through the recovery process and treatment plan continuum, his or her ability to feel confidence and control his or her symptoms often is guided by available resources, absence of substance use disorders, and motivation to stay in treatment.

Psychosocial recovery and rehabilitation are key aspects that foster successful treatment outcomes and community integration, and improve functional outcomes, independence, symptomatic remission, meaningful relationships, and quality of life. Psychiatric nurses have vital responsibilities and opportunities to help the patient attain these goals.

## SUMMARY

Psychiatric nurses are poised to establish meaningful relationships with patients and their families as they face the challenges of coping with severe and chronic psychiatric disorders. One example of a psychosocial recovery and rehabilitation model uses an intensive case management approach. This approach offers an interdisciplinary model that integrates pharmacotherapy, social cognition training, cognitive remediation, and family involvement. This evidence-based plan of care instills hope and nurtures one's capacity to learn and improve function and quality of life. It is cost-effective and offers psychiatric nurses opportunities to facilitate symptom remission, facilitate self-efficacy, and improve communication and social cognition. Ultimately, nursing interventions promote a higher level of functioning and quality of life. Nurses in diverse practice settings must be willing to plan and implement innovative treatment models that provide seamless mental health care across the mental health treatment continuum.

## REFERENCES

1. Drake RE, Goldman HH, Leff HS, et al. Implementing evidence-based practices in routine mental health service settings. Psychiatr Serv 2001;52:179–82.
2. President's New Freedom Commission on Mental Health. Achieving the promise: transforming mental health care in America—executive summary. 2003. Available at: http://store.samhsa.gov/product/Achieving-the-Promise-Transforming-Mental-Health-Care-in-America-Executive-Summary/SMA03-3831. Accessed October 12, 2015.
3. United States Public Health Service Office of the Surgeon General. Mental health: culture, race, and ethnicity: a supplement to mental health: a report of the surgeon general. Rockville (MD): Department of Health and Human Services; U.S. Public Health Service; 2001.
4. Substance Abuse and Mental Health Services Administration. Leading change: a plan for SAMHSA's roles and actions 2011-2014 executive summary and introduction. Rockville (MD): Substance Abuse and Mental Health Services Administration; 2011. HHS publication No. (SMA) 11-4629 summary.
5. Gaumond P, Whitter M. Access to recovery (ATR) approaches to recovery-oriented systems of care: three case studies. Rockville (MD): Center for Substance Abuse Treatment; Substance Abuse and Mental Health Services Administration; 2009. HHS publication No. (SMA) 09–4440. Available at: http://www.samhsa.gov/sites/default/files/partnersforrecovery/docs/ATR_Approaches_to_ROSC.pdf. Accessed October 26, 2015.
6. Painter K. Evidence-based practices in community mental health: outcome evaluation. J Behav Health Serv Res 2012;39:434–44.

7. Chinman M, George P, Dougherty RH, et al. Peer support services for individuals with serious mental illnesses: assessing the evidence. Psychiatr Serv 2014;65: 429–41.

8. Chinman M, Young AS, Hassell J, et al. Toward the implementation of mental health consumer provider services. J Behav Health Serv Res 2006;33:176–95.

9. Corrigan PW, Slopen N, Gracia G, et al. Some recovery processes in mutual-help groups for persons with mental illness. II: Qualitative analysis of participant interviews. Community Ment Health J 2005;2005(41):721–35.

10. Coniglio FD, Hancock N, Ellis LA. Peer support within clubhouse: a grounded theory study. Community Ment Health J 2012;48:153–60.

11. Valencia M, Fresan A, Barak Y, et al. Predicting functional remission in patients with schizophrenia: a cross-sectional study of symptomatic remission, psychosocial remission, functioning, and clinical outcome. Neuropsychiatr Dis Treat 2015; 11:2339–48.

12. Brewer WJ, Lambert TJ, Witt K, et al. Intensive case management for high-risk patients with first-episode psychosis: service model and outcomes. Lancet Psychiatry 2015;2:29–37.

13. Robinson D, Gallego J, John M, et al. Psychosis prevention: a randomized comparison of aripiprazole and risperidone for the acute treatment of first-episode schizophrenia and related disorders: 3-month outcomes. Schizophr Bull 2015; 41(6):1227–36.

14. Nakajima S, Takeuchi H, Fervaha G, et al. Comparative efficacy between clozapine and other atypical antipsychotics on depressive symptoms in patients with schizophrenia: analysis of the CATIE phase 2E data. Schizophr Res 2015; 161:429–33.

15. Galderisi S, Merlotti E, Mucci A. Neurobiological background of negative symptoms. Eur Arch Psychiatry Clin Neurosci 2015;2015(7):543–58.

16. Dhillon AS, Dollieslager LP. Rehab rounds: overcoming barriers to individualized psychosocial rehabilitation in an acute treatment unit of a state hospital. Psychiatr Serv 2000;51:313–7.

17. Mueser KT, Bond GR, Drake RE, et al. Model in community care for severe mental illness: a review of research on case management. Schizophr Bull 1998;24: 37–74.

18. Hengartner MP, Klauser M, Heim G, et al. Introduction of a psychosocial post-discharge intervention program aimed at reducing psychiatric rehospitalization rates and at improving mental health and functioning. Perspect Psychiatr Care 2015. http://dx.doi.org/10.1111/ppc.12131.

19. Marshall M, Lockwood A. WITHDRAWN: assertive community treatment for people with severe mental disorders. Cochrane Database Syst Rev 2011;(4):CD001089.

20. Warren BJ. Home and community-based care. In: Antai-Otong D, editor. Psychiatric mental health nursing: behavioral and biological concepts. Clifton Park (NY): Delmar Learning; 2008. p. 1005–23.

21. Revell ER, Neill JC, Harte M, et al. A systematic review and meta-analysis of cognitive remediation in early schizophrenia. Schizophr Res 2015;168:213–22.

22. Harvey PD. What is the evidence for changes in cognition and functioning over the lifespan in patients with schizophrenia? J Clin Psychiatry 2014;75(Suppl 2): 34–8.

23. Bellack A, Mueser K. Psychosocial treatment of schizophrenia. Schizophr Bull 1993;19:317–36.

24. Atadokht A, Hajloo N, Karimi M, et al. The role of family expressed emotion and perceived social support in predicting addiction relapse. Int J High Risk Behav Addict 2015;4(1):e21250, eCollection 2015.
25. Koutra K, Triljva S, Roumeliotaki T, et al. Impaired family functioning in psychosis and its relevance to relapse: a two-year follow-up study. Compr Psychiatry 2015; 62:1–12.
26. Birchwood M, Todd P, Jackson C. Early intervention in psychosis: a critical period hypothesis. Br J Psychiatry 1998;172(Suppl 33):53–9.
27. Lutgens D, Iver S, Jooper R, et al. A five-year randomized parallel and blinded clinical trial of an extended specialized early intervention vs. regular care in the early phase of psychotic disorders: study protocol. BMC Psychiatry 2015;15:22.
28. Windell DL, Norman R, Lal S, et al. Subjective experiences of illness recovery in individuals treated for first-episode psychosis. Soc Psychiatry Psychiatr Epidemiol 2015;50:1069–77.
29. Anderson CM, Reiss DJ, Hogarty GE. Schizophrenia and the family: a practitioner's guide to psychoeducation and management. New York: Guilford Press; 1986.
30. Kinoshita Y, Furukawa TA, Kinoshita K, et al. Supported employment for adults with severe mental illness. Cochrane Database Syst Rev 2013;(9):CD008297.
31. Ng SS, Lak DC, Lee SC, et al. Concurrent validation of a neurocognitive assessment protocol for clients with mental illness in job matching as shop sales in supported employment. East Asian Arch Psychiatry 2015;25:21–8.

# Evidence-Based Care of the Patient with Borderline Personality Disorder

Deborah Antai-Otong, MS, APRN, PMHCNS-BC, FAAN

KEYWORDS

- Borderline personality disorder • Nonsuicidal self-injury (NSSI) • Parasuicide
- Impulsivity • Dialectal behavioral therapy • Mentalization-CBT • Attachment theory

KEY POINTS

- It is important to examine major underpinnings of borderline personality disorder (BPD).
- There are many nursing implications for caring for patients with BPD.
- It is vital to assess suicide risk factors and self-injurious behaviors in patients with BPD.
- There are evidence-based pharmacologic and psychotherapeutic approaches used in the treatment of BPD.

## INTRODUCTION

Borderline personality disorder (BPD) refers to a personality disorder whose primary symptoms include significant emotional distress, striking impulsivity, and impairment of interpersonal and occupational functioning or both.[1] The age of onset varies, but it often ranges from adolescence to early adulthood (ages 18–25 years). Typically the patient with BPD has marked reactions to rejection and abandonment, chaotic patterns of interpersonal relationships, unstable mood and self-image disturbances, self-harm behaviors, and other maladaptive coping behaviors.[1–3] Major concerns of nurses and other health providers involve the high use of health care resources among patients with BPD normally arising from suicide attempts and other self-harm and demanding behaviors.

The precise prevalence of BPD is obscure, but estimates are about 2% in community samples and 6% in primary care populations, and approximately 15% to 20% of patients seen in outpatient mental health settings.[1,3,4] Severity of symptoms may vary from moderately disabling to severely incapacitating. A large percentage of patients

---

This article is an update of an article previously published in *Nursing Clinics of North America*, Volume 38, Issue 1, March 2003.

The author has no financial interests to disclose.

Department of Veterans Affairs, Veterans Integrated Service Networks-(VISN-17), 2301 E. Lamar Boulevard, Arlington, TX 76006, USA

*E-mail address:* Deborah.Antai-Otong@va.gov

with BPD, approximately 75%, have a history of self-harm or deliberate nonsuicidal self-injury (NSSI) and 10% lifetime risk of completed suicides.[2,4] BPD is like to co-occur with other psychiatric conditions, including anxiety disorders, major depressive disorders, eating disorders, and substance use disorders and medical conditions (eg, somatization disorders, chronic pain disorder). Estimates indicate that 75% of patients diagnosed with BPD are women.[1,4–6]

A major challenge confronting nurses and other health care providers is the high suicidality and other self-harm behaviors among patients with BPD. One in 10 patients with BPD completes suicide, but suicide is readily preventable, and it does not necessarily occur during treatment.[2,4] Chronic suicidal behavior is best understood as a barometer of the patient's level of distress and ability to modulate negative emotions. Hospitalization has not been shown to reduce suicide and often has negative results. Community studies have shown that the rates of suicide peak between the ages of 18 and 30 and decrease with age.[2–4,7] The highest risk of suicide among patients with BPD occurs in those with co-occurring substance use disorders and mood disorders and histories of past attempts. Normally, patients presenting with acute suicidality also meet criteria for depressive illness. In comparison, patients presenting with chronic suicidal ideations are seeking treatment.[8]

Because patients with BPD are high users of health care resources, most nurses have had contact with these patients. The patient with BPD often challenges the patience of nurses, hence, the risk of rejection and poor treatment outcomes. This article focuses on strategies that can improve therapeutic environments that convey empathy, establish clear and health boundaries, and facilitate appropriate limit settings and an optimal level of functioning. Finally, this article provides an overview of the complexity of this challenging personality disorder, causative factors, assessment and diagnostic considerations, and person-centered and interdisciplinary treatment.

## CAUSATIVE FACTORS

A large body of research suggests that BPD is a problem arising from numerous factors, such as trauma or abuse, genetic predisposition, and dysregulations of neurobiologic processes.[9–11] Of particular interest is the relationship between causative factors and self-injurious behaviors. Numerous data indicate a host of biologic correlates of suicidal and other self-injurious behaviors related to decreased levels of serotonin (5-hydroxytryptamine) found in the brainstems of suicide victims and lows levels of cerebrospinal fluid 5-hydroxyindolaecetic acid found in attempters.[11,12] A plethora of data also supports the assumption that underpinnings of BPD arise from dysregulation of the prefrontal cortex, which is the focal point of self-direction, self-organization, and emotional regulation.[13] These data also indicate the importance of diverse treatment interventions, comprising pharmacologic and nonpharmacologic interventions, to treat this complex psychiatric disorder.

## ASSESSMENT AND DIAGNOSTIC CONSIDERATIONS

Typically the patient seeks treatment during a perceived crisis that parallels a real or imagined valued relationship breakup. Patients with BPD have difficulty being alone, and relationship breakups worsen their anxiety and distress. Mood swings are common, resulting in a dysphoric or depressed mood later. Their clinging or "smothering" behaviors tend to generate various emotions in nurses. During these periods, the nurse must convey empathy, maintain clear and consistent boundaries, explain all procedures, and work with other providers to maintain consistent and firm limit setting. Intense negative emotional states challenge nurses to control their own negative reactions and form therapeutic interactions.

Establishing a therapeutic relationship entails conveying empathy and concern, while maintaining clear boundaries. The nurse has an opportunity to *recognize* personal boundaries between self and patients. Nurses must define their role as a health care provider and not a "buddy or friend." A failure to do so increases the risk of blurred boundaries and confusion in the patient's expectations from the nurse and relationship. Patients with BPD are experts at determining and "pushing" the nurse's "buttons." An example of "pushing buttons" may be seen when the patient makes personal attacks about the nurse's appearance or questioning his or her educational preparation. It behooves the nurse to recognize these behaviors as maladaptive interpersonal features of BPD and to refrain from responding defensively or angrily. Nurses must focus on the issues at hand by making statements such as, "Mary, what does the size of my hips or my educational preparation have to do with our discussion concerning your behavior?" A failure to understand one's own "buttons" increases the risk of reinforcing negative and rejecting responses to the patient, who ironically, needs empathy and understanding.

Another important aspect of the assessment process includes making a differential diagnosis of medical conditions, substance use disorder, or psychiatric conditions and performing a mental status examination. Major components of a mental status examination are listed in **Box 1**.

Suicidal assessment includes questions about present thoughts, plan, means, intent, and imminence of acting on thoughts/plans; past suicide attempts; and other self-injurious or self-harm behaviors (eg, cutting, burning). Growing evidence indicates that individuals with BPD report a history of deliberate NSSI, particularly among adolescents and adults with co-occurring depression or anxiety disorders and BPD.[13] NSSI refers to a purposeful and self-inflicted destruction of body tissue without the wish to die. Functions of NSSI behaviors vary, but most research indicates an absence of pain during the episode and that it seems to act as a dissociative defense (ie, depersonalization and perceptual distortions) or to activate the release of the brain's pain-reward-processing neural pathways.[14,15]

The above-listed data must be documented and discussed with various members of the treatment team. When a differential diagnosis is made, thus ruling out medical,

---

**Box 1**
**Major components of a mental status examination**

- Chief complaint or reasons for seeking treatment
- Current and previous coping skills related to crises
- Quality of support systems, including current relationships, employment, finances
- General appearance, including the mode of arrival, cooperativeness, and eye contact (consider cultural factors)
- Mood and affect
- Speech that includes rate, quality, and clarity
- Thought content and processes
- Sensorium and other higher brain function, including memory, judgment, reliability, and insight into present illness (crisis) and treatment
- Level of dangerousness to self and others

psychiatric, and substance-use disorders, the nurse and other team members can determine if the patient has BPD.

The essential features of a patient with BPD include the following:

- A pervasive pattern of intense chaotic or unstable interpersonal relationships
- Marked emotional distress and lability
- Intense fears of abandonment
- Low self-esteem
- Marked identity disturbances
- Hypersensitivity to object loss
- Intolerance of being alone
- Chronic dysphoria (intense sadness and other negative emotions)
- Intense anger and rage
- Chronic history of impulsivity and mood instability
- Chronic feelings of emptiness and lack of nurturing and support
- Recurrent maladaptive coping responses, including self-harm behaviors
- Transient, stress-induced delusional ideation, or intense and brief dissociative reactions[1-4]

It is imperative for the nurse to recognize that BPD is an axis II disorder (personality disorder) and to recognize the high co-occurrence of depression, anxiety disorders, and substance use disorders (axis I). There is overwhelming evidence that links axis I disorders with BPD because of early childhood traumas and adversities. These disorders must be assessed and treated appropriately. A failure to assess axis I diagnoses increases the risk of suicide and other self-harm behaviors. The following discussion describes how the patient with BPD may present in primary care settings and emergency departments.

In primary care and other practice settings, the patient may go from one provider to another with various somatic and psychiatric complaints, generating chaos and "staff splitting," which result in anger and frustration and a failure to address the patient's concerns appropriately.[16,17] These patients are sometimes referred to as "difficult patients." Nurses must maintain an empathetic and accepting demeanor and set firm and consistent limits with the demanding patient. Despite the tendency to focus on somatic complaints, these symptoms require a thorough physical evaluation. Because of patients' intense dependency needs and hostility toward staff when staff fails to meet them in a timely manner, nurses must anticipate intense rage and anger and respond appropriately and assertively.

An assessment and diagnostic feature of BPD is suicidality and other self-harm behaviors. Nurses in various mental health settings need to accept these symptoms and focus on treatment planning on dealing with underlying causes. It is imperative for the nurse to respond emphatically rather than judgmentally, while assessing the patient's imminent risk of danger to self or others. When a patient attempts suicide, it is imperative to avoid reinforcing this behavior, but rather to strengthen adaptive coping behaviors. The level of care necessary after an attempt parallels the seriousness or lethality of the attempt. Often the patient threatens suicide or other self-harm behaviors, and the patient must be taken seriously and assessed and managed appropriately. When caring for the patient with BPD who expresses suicidal intent, a failure to misjudge the risk may be tragic.

Patients with BPD are likely to have a different presentation when they arrive in emergency departments than primary care settings. During a psychiatric crisis, the patient may be overdosed, may have cut a wrist, or may exhibit self-destructive behaviors or threats. Because of the high risk of self-harm, nursing staff must search carefully for sharp objects, illicit and licit medications, and other harmful items. Major goals in the emergency department include harm-prevention, medical and psychiatric stabilization, and addressing the patient's emotional and psychiatric needs. Nurses must convey concern and provide consistent and firm limit setting during a psychiatric emergency.[18] When the patient is medically cleared, psychiatric interventions can be implemented. Additional treatment considerations during a psychiatric emergency include verbal de-escalation, pharmacologic interventions, and other psychotherapeutic interventions. When the patient's emotional and psychiatric conditions are stable, the nurse and other team members must make an appropriate mental health referral and disposition. An in-depth discussion of specific pharmacotherapy and psychotherapeutic approaches follows in later discussion.

Normally the patient is involved in a treatment program with a team or primary therapist. The central role of the primary therapist is to oversee safety and contract for safety and hospitalization if necessary to stabilize acute medical and psychiatric conditions. Contacting the therapist is helpful in validating information and ensuring adequate follow-up. If the patient is not in treatment, consultation with a mental health professional or center is crucial to ensure appropriate and timely follow-up. A "no-harm" or safety contract is necessary during a crisis situation to avail options to the patient and family in the event of recurrent suicidal thoughts and imminent danger to self or others with a caveat that the merits of this intervention are questionable.[19] Safety contracts, which lack empirical support for the effectiveness concerning in the prevention of suicide, do not replace a comprehensive suicide risk assessment because overreliance on them may jeopardize the patient's safety and suicide risk.[19]

Likewise, suicide assessment scales have little prognostic value and are unreliable in forecasting suicide. Contracting for safety often includes the following:

- Ask the patient to give explicit agreement not harm him or herself
- Generate a safety plan with written and verbal instructions of what to do in the event of recurrent and imminent thoughts (eg, close friend/family member, suicide crisis line, 911)
- Inquire about access to firearms
- Reinforce the responsibility of safety to the patient and not the nurse to work out with others during a crisis situation
- Collaborate with family members or friends who may help to resolve the crisis
- Make appropriate mental health referrals and schedule follow-up[18]
- *Screen all* patients for suicidal risk during initial contact and remain alert to this issue throughout assessment process.

Thorough documentation of the decision-making process is crucial. Although hospitalization may be considered, as a result of primary care guidelines, certain parameters have been established that support hospitalization (ie, imminent danger to self or others, unstable psychiatric and medical conditions). A plethora of research indicates that hospitalization is unproven to be effective in the prevention of suicide, and it has limited indications. Specific indications for acute psychiatric hospitalization of the patient with BPD include transient stress-induced psychosis, life-threatening suicide attempts, and NSSI behaviors.[20] Sometimes a brief hospitalization enables the interdisciplinary treatment team to review treatment planning and allows for medication stabilization. Negative consequences of hospitalization include dependency and reinforcement of maladaptive behaviors.

An important point to remember about the patient at risk for suicide is assessing the level of the nurse involvement. Specifically, nurses must refrain from "rescuing" or "rejecting" the patient who threatens suicide and focus more on assessing the need for involvement behind the thoughts and threats (**Box 2**).

## PHARMACOLOGIC AND PSYCHOTHERAPEUTIC CONSIDERATIONS

Because of the complexity of BPD and continual risk of suicide, nurses must enlist a person-centered, strength-based intervention and interdisciplinary approach to facilitate adaptive coping skills and optimal level of functioning. Depending on the nurse's educational preparation and clinical expertise, the nurse is likely to provide an array of mental health services. Likely mental health services often comprise medication administration or management, psychoeducation, intensive case management, and various psychotherapies. Nurses in primary care settings and other non-mental health settings must collaborate with mental health nurses and other mental health professionals to avoid becoming part of the "splitting" behaviors, which are common in patients with BPD. These behaviors generate tension and interpersonal conflicts between staff and interfere with optimizing treatment modalities. Pharmacologic and psychotherapeutic interventions are key components of treatment planning and have proven efficacy in helping patients cope with intense emotional states, dysphoria (intense sadness), and impulsivity or dyscontrol behaviors.

### Pharmacologic Interventions

Prevailing evidence indicates that the treatment of BPD necessitates a comprehensive, person-centered, holistic, and long treatment (ie, psychotherapy and symptom-targeted adjunctive pharmacotherapy).[21,22]

Pharmacologic treatment is frequently used to treat BPD, although there are no practice guidelines that recommend or approve of use to treat this disorder. Most pharmacologic interventions are symptom specific.[23,24] Target symptoms for pharmacologic interventions of patients with BPD include 3 dimensions: cognitive-perceptual disturbances, affective lability, and impulsive-behavior dyscontrol behaviors. Growing evidence reveals that antidepressants, mood-stabilizing anticonvulsants (ie, valproate acid), and atypical antipsychotics (ie, quetiapine) improve core symptoms of BPD, but they are not a cure-all.[23,24] Based on prevailing evidence, pharmacologic agents are not recommended first-line treatment for BPD and are used as an adjunctive treatment with psychotherapeutic approaches.

Cognitive-perceptual disturbances include transient stress-induced psychosis, paranoia, suspiciousness, distrust, dissociation, and illusions. Management of these

---

**Box 2**
**How to assess for suicide risk**

- *Establish* rapport and provide a supportive nonjudgmental environment
- *Ensure* safety—remove sharps and other dangerous items and secure belongings
- Keep questions simple, clear, and direct
- Use open-ended questions
- Assess for level of lethality (eg, increased risk with a highly specific plan, means, previous attempts, previously rehearsed)
- *Never leave a person at risk for suicide alone*
- *Do not promise* the person threatening suicide that you will keep this information confidential

symptoms includes low-dose and short-term atypical antipsychotic medications, such as olanzapine and aripiprazole.[23,24] Implications for nurses include assessing for adverse side effects, such as sedation, significant weight gain, extrapyramidal side effects, and other movement disorders associated with antipsychotic medications. Despite the high use of these agents, studies fail to demonstrate consistent evidence of their efficacy in the treatment of BPD.

Symptoms of *affective instability* or mood disturbances include depressed or irritable mood and loss of interest in activities that were once considered pleasurable. Historically, antidepressants, such as selective serotonin re-uptake inhibitors, have been considered first-line treatment partly because they were also effective in the treatment of co-occurring disorders, such as anxiety disorders and aggression, irritability, and NSSI behaviors.[23,24] Some researchers suggest that antidepressants cannot be considered first-line treatment because they fail to demonstrate efficacy in managing impulsive-dyscontrol behaviors.[23,24]

*Impulsive-behavioral dyscontrol* consists of self-harm behaviors, such as parasuicides, aggressiveness, substance use, and NSSI (eg, self-cutting, self-burning). In addition to antidepressants, other medications with proven efficacy include anticonvulsant agents, lithium, and anxiolytic medications.[20–23]

### Social Cognitive Disturbances

Researchers submit that individuals with BPD have social cognitive disturbances related to dysregulation of mentalization and that this concept contributes to the core symptoms of BPD (eg, emotional dysregulation, NSSI).[25–27] Purportedly, patients with BPD have impaired mentalization that stems from a failure to form early childhood attachments or healthy relationships with primary caregivers and neurologic and psychological development.[25–27] Healthy relationships with primary caregivers are critical in the development of these important processes that underlie mentalization, positive self-esteem and self-image, modulation of stress and impulse control, and healthy relationships across the lifespan. *Mentalization* is an ability to accurately appraise one's emotional states and subsequent psychological and behavioral responses and those in others. It also helps individuals to discern how their own behavior affects others.[25–27] Growing evidence indicates that insecure attachments increase the risk of BPD and other psychiatric conditions. This premise has indications for psychotherapeutic interventions.

Symptom management is multifaceted and is determined by the patient's present symptoms, wishes, preferences, and individual needs. Poorer clinical outcomes are associated with the quality of early childhood primary caregiver (eg, infant-mother) attachments, coexisting substance-use disorder, and severity of early childhood adversities.[2,3,5] Bowlby's attachment theory[28] is based on the quality of relationships with early childhood caregivers and healthy development. These relationships provide the basis of lifelong interpersonal and intrapersonal interactions. Most studies indicate a person-centered approach that integrates pharmacologic and psychotherapeutic interventions is the most effective. This plan of care must identify clearly the primary psychotherapist, identify a plan to respond to crisis, and monitor the patient's safety and coordination of treatment planning by an interdisciplinary team.[22,29]

### Psychotherapeutic Interventions

Psychotherapeutic interventions are considered the primary approach for treating patients with BPD. The decision to use specific psychotherapeutic interventions depends on the patient's clinical presentation and preferences. Poor treatment candidates are patients who exhibit severe antisocial behaviors and coexisting substance use disorders. Additional prognostic factors include adherence to treatment and reducing high-risk behaviors, such as high intelligence, a lack of early childhood abuse, and a lack of co-occurring substance use disorders.[29–31]

Studies reveal growing promise in the treatment of BPD using cognitive and behavioral interventions.[25,27,29–31] Dialectical behavior is a cognitive behavioral model that entails active and structured work to analyze and modify target behaviors through cognitive restructuring, skills training, exposure techniques, and a contingency plan. The premise behind this treatment modality is that persons with BPD lack the capacity to modulate emotions or feelings. An inability to regulate emotions is reinforced by a continuous transaction between the patient's emotional vulnerabilities and external world of invalidation. This approach involves 3 concurrent modes of treatment: weekly individual sessions, a weekly group specifically for skills training, and telephone contacts by the primary nurse psychotherapist on an as-needed basis.[29]

Psychodynamic psychotherapy also is being used to treat BPD. Compared with dialectical behavior therapy, this approach enables the nurse psychotherapist to explore patterns of feelings and underlying behaviors. This treatment modality also involves individual psychotherapy and group therapy that focuses on skills training. Mentalizing-based treatment has been introduced in the treatment of BPD.[25–27] This approach helps the patient make sense of his or her own and others' personal emotional affect regulation and self-identity with the goal of improving interpersonal relationships and social functioning.

## SUMMARY

BPD is a serious and cost-consuming psychiatric disorder. The high prevalence of patients with BPD and co-occurring depression, eating disorders, and substance-use disorders in primary care and mental health settings contributes to their high use of resources in these practice settings. Recurrent suicidal behaviors and threats and NSSI behaviors increase demands on nurses and other health care providers. Regardless of treatment challenges associated with BPD, researchers suggest a more positive outlook in the treatment of this complex psychiatric condition. Nurses must be able to interact with individuals with BPD by using an empathetic and unbiased approach while maintaining healthy boundaries. This article has focused on areas in which nurses can understand major underpinnings of BPD; assess their client's immediate needs; and initiate evidence-based strategies to resolve distressful emotional states and self-injurious behaviors.

## REFERENCES

1. American Psychiatric Association. Diagnostic and statistical manual of mental disorders. 5th edition. Washington, DC: Author; 2013.
2. Gunderson JG, Links P. Borderline personality disorder: a clinical guide. 2nd edition. Washington, DC: American Psychiatric Publishing; 2008.
3. Gunderson JG. Reducing suicide risk in borderline personality disorder. JAMA 2015;314:181–2.
4. Gunderson JG. Clinical practice: borderline personality disorder. N Engl J Med 2011;364:2037–42.
5. Paris J. Treatment of borderline personality disorder: a guide to evidence-based practice. New York: Guilford Press; 2008.
6. Campbell G, Bruno R, Darke S, et al. Associations of borderline personality with pain, problems with medications and suicidality in a community sample of

chronic non-cancer pain patients prescribed opioids for pain. Gen Hosp Psychiatry 2015;37:434–40.

7. Cooper LD, Balsis S, Oltmanns TF. Aging: empirical contribution. A longitudinal analysis of personality disorder dimensions and personality traits in a community sample of older adults: perspectives from selves and informants. J Pers Disord 2014;28:151–65.

8. Dixon-Gordon KL, Weiss NH, Tull MT, et al. Characterizing emotional dysfunction in borderline personality, major depression, and their co-occurrence. Compr Psychiatry 2015;62:187–203.

9. O'Neill A, D'Souza A, Samson AC, et al. Dysregulation between emotion and theory of mind networks in borderline personality disorder. Psychiatry Res 2015;231:25–32.

10. Cullen KR, LaRiviere LL, Vizueta N, et al. Brain activation in response to overt and covert fear and happy faces in women with borderline personality disorder. Brain Imaging Behav 2015. [Epub ahead of print].

11. Coccaro EF, Fanning JR, Phan KL, et al. Serotonin and impulsive aggression. CNS Spectr 2015;231:25–32.

12. Sullivan GM, Oquendo MA, Milak M, et al. Positron emission tomography quantification of serotonin (1A) receptor binding in suicide attempters with major depressive disorder. JAMA Psychiatry 2015;72:169–78.

13. Groschwitz RC, Plener PL, Kaess, et al. The situation of former adolescent self-injurers as young adults: a follow-up study. BMC Psychiatry 2015;15:160.

14. Borges LM, Naugle AE. An experimental examination of the interaction between mood induction task and personality psychopathology on state emotion dysregulation. Behav Sci (Basel) 2015;9:70–92.

15. Osuch E, Ford K, Wrath A, et al. Functional MRI of pain application in youth who engaged in repetitive non-suicidal self-injury vs. psychiatric controls. Psychiatry Res 2014;223:104–12.

16. Sansone RA, Dittoe N, Halm HS, et al. The prevalence of borderline personality disorder in a consecutive sample of cardiac stress test patients. Prim Care Companion CNS Disord 2011;13(3):e1–2.

17. Sansone RA, Sansone LA. Borderline personality disorder in the medical setting: suggestive behaviors, syndromes, and diagnoses. Innov Clin Neurosci 2015;12:39–44.

18. Antai-Otong D. Psychiatric emergencies: how to accurately assess and manage the patient in crisis. Eau Claire (WI): PESI; 2009.

19. Garvey KA, Penn JV, Campbell AL, et al. Contracting for safety with patients: clinical practice and forensic implications. J Am Acad Psychiatry Law 2009;37:363–70.

20. Nelson KJ. Managing borderline personality disorder on general psychiatric units. Psychodyn Psychiatry 2013;41:563–74.

21. National Collaborating Centre for Mental Health. Borderline personality disorder: treatment and management. Full Guideline. Clinical Guideline 78. Manchester (UK): NICE; 2009. Available at: http://www.nice.org.uk/nicemedia/pdf/CG78FullGuideline.pdf. Accessed October 2, 2015.

22. Vita A, De Peri L, Sachetti E. Antipsychotics, antidepressants, anticonvulsants, and placebo on the symptom dimensions of borderline personality disorder: a meta-analysis of randomized controlled and open-label trials. J Clin Psychopharmacol 2011;31:613–24.

23. Bridler R, Haberle A, Muller ST, et al. Psychopharmacological treatment of 2195 in-patients with borderline personality disorder: a comparison with other psychiatric disorders. Eur Neuropsychopharmacol 2015;25:763–72.

24. Zanarini MC, Frankenburg DB, Fitzmaurice G. Attainment and stability of sustained symptomatic remission and recovery among patients with borderline personality disorder and axis II comparison subjects: a 16-year prospective follow-up study. Am J Psychiatry 2012;169:476–83.

25. Bateman A, Fonagy P. Mentalization based treatment for borderline personality disorder. World Psychiatry 2010;9:11–5.

26. Fonagy P, Bateman A. The development of borderline personality disorder–a mentalizing model. J Pers Disord 2008;22:4–21.

27. Bateman A, Fonagy P. Randomized controlled trial of outpatient mentalization-based treatment versus structured clinical management for borderline personality disorder. Am J Psychiatry 2009;166:1355–64.

28. Bowlby J. A secure base: parent-child attachment and healthy human development. New York: Basic Books; 1988.

29. Linehan MM, Korslund KE, Harned MS, et al. Dialectical behavior therapy for high suicide risk in individuals with borderline personality disorder: a randomized clinical trial and component analysis. JAMA Psychiatry 2015;72:475–82.

30. Stoffers JM, Vollm BA, Rucker G, et al. Psychological therapies for people with borderline personality disorder. Cochrane Database Syst Rev 2012;(8):CD005652.

31. Andreasson K, Krogh J, Rosenbaum B, et al. The DiaS trial: dialectical behavior therapy versus collaborative assessment and management of suicidality on self-harm in patients with a recent suicide attempt and borderline personality disorder traits—study protocol for a randomized controlled trial. Trials 2014;15:194.

# Adverse Drug Reactions Associated with Antipsychotics, Antidepressants, Mood Stabilizers, and Stimulants

Courtney J. Givens, PharmD

## KEYWORDS

- Side effects • Adverse drug reactions • Psychotropic medications
- Movement disorders

## KEY POINTS

- Side effects (SEs) and adverse drug reactions (ADRs) contribute to medication noncompliance, morbidity, and mortality.
- Many ADRs may be prevented and common SEs can be managed.
- Patient safety and medication compliance are essential components of psychiatric care; therefore, nursing interventions that prevent or resolve SEs/ADRs are important.

The advent of psychotropic medications in the 1950s greatly impacted the practice of psychiatry. Since then, efforts have been made to produce effective medications with few SEs or ADRs. Newer psychotropic medications have been developed, thus offering treatment options with more favorable SE profiles, but, despite these advancements, patients taking psychotropic medications still experience SEs or ADRs.

An ADR is defined as a response to a medication that is noxious, unintended, and may occur at normal therapeutic doses.[1,2] An SE is any undesirable secondary effect of a medication outside its intended therapeutic action.[3] ADRs can lead to morbidity and mortality and are currently ranked as the fourth leading cause of death in the United States following heart disease, cancer, and stroke.[4] Therefore, addressing psychotropic-related ADRs is an important component of improving patient safety and quality of life. In many cases ADRs can be prevented through appropriate

This article is an update of an article previously published in Nursing Clinics of North America, Volume 38, Issue 1, March 2003.
Disclosures: None.
Mental Health, VA North Texas Health Care System, 4500 South Lancaster Road, Dallas, TX 75216, USA
E-mail address: Courtney.Givens@VA.gov

monitoring and prescribing practices. Health care providers should always be vigilant in patients with increased risk of ADRs. Factors shown to increase the risk of ADRs include[5]

- Polypharmacy
- Multiple comorbidities
- Substance use disorders
- Renal or hepatic impairment
- Young or advanced age

Furthermore, ADRs and SEs are frequently implicated in nonadherence to psychotropic medications. A study of patients with schizophrenia found 86.19% of the population experienced at least 1 antipsychotic-related SE, and SEs were linked to significantly lower rates of medication adherence.[6] Adherence to pharmacotherapy is an important aspect of treatment; therefore, nursing interventions that identify, prevent, and manage SEs and ADRs are crucial in psychiatric practice. This article discusses ADRs and SEs as well as interventions associated with 4 psychotropic drug classes.

## PSYCHOTROPIC MEDICATIONS

Psychotropic medications are generally classified based on target symptoms, mechanisms of action, and SE profile. The drug categories discussed in this article as well as the corresponding diseases states they typically treat are listed in **Table 1**. Conventional antidepressants, such as monoamine oxidase inhibitors (MAOIs) and tricyclic antidepressants (TCAs), are not discussed.

## ANTIPSYCHOTIC OR NEUROLEPTIC AGENTS

Antipsychotic or neuroleptic agents are most commonly prescribed for psychosis but also may be prescribed for treatment refractory depression, bipolar depression, and mania. Antipsychotics have been used to treat behavioral symptoms of dementia but should be avoided due to a black box warning for increased risk of death when antipsychotics are used for this indication. There is variability between individual antipsychotic agents' SE profiles, but antipsychotics can be grouped into 2 classes, first-generation/conventional antipsychotics and second-generation/atypical antipsychotics (**Box 1** and **Table 2**). Common SEs among antipsychotics include sedation, weight gain, hypotension, sexual dysfunction, and anticholinergic effects.[7] See **Table 4** for more information on management. When choosing an antipsychotic agent, one goal is avoiding SEs; therefore, understanding SE profiles is important.

| Table 1 Psychotropic drug classes | |
|---|---|
| **Drug Class** | **Disease State** |
| Antipsychotic or neuroleptic agents | Psychotics disorders, schizophrenia, mania, substance-induced psychosis, or treatment-resistant depression |
| Antidepressants | Depression and anxiety |
| Mood stabilizers | Bipolar disorder and other mood disorders |
| Stimulants | Attention-deficit/hyperactivity disorder |

| Box 1<br>Second-generation or atypical antipsychotics |
| --- |
| Aripiprazole (Abilify) |
| Clozapine (Clozaril) |
| Iloperidone (Fanapt) |
| Ziprasidone (Geodon) |
| Paliperidone (Invega) |
| Lurasidone (Latuda) |
| Brexpiprazole (Rexulti) |
| Risperidone (Risperdal) |
| Quetiapine (Seroquel) |
| Asenapine (Saphris) |
| Olanzapine (Zyprexa) |

## First-generation (or Conventional) Antipsychotics

### Movement disorders

First-generation antipsychotics (FGAs) work primarily through blockade of the dopamine ($D_2$) receptor at varying potencies. Blockade of $D_2$ receptors in the mesolimbic $D_2$ pathway results in the therapeutic effects of antipsychotics. Blockade in other pathways, however, may lead to SEs. For example, $D_2$ blockade in the nigrostriatal pathway results in one of the most common concerns during treatment with FGAs, movement abnormalities. This risk of movement disorders is highest with high-potency FGAs. Antipsychotic-induced movement disorders include akathisia, acute dystonia, tardive dyskinesia, and drug-induced parkinsonism.[8] Second-generation antipsychotics (SGAs) may cause movement disorders, but the risk is lower compared with high-potency FGAs. Assessment scales, such as the Abnormal Involuntary Movement Scale and Barnes Akathisia Rating Scale, are available to assess movement abnormalities. Nursing interventions are important in addressing movement abnormalities, which can be distressing and debilitating.

Description and management of antipsychotic-induced movement abnormalities[7–9]:

Akathisia: feeling of inner restlessness resulting in leg movements, pacing, fidgeting, and/or intense anxiety. It usually occurs within the first 3 months of antipsychotic treatment but may occur at any time. Management includes antipsychotic dose reduction, if possible; β-blockers (propranolol); or benzodiazepines.

Acute dystonia: acute spasms of any muscle in the body but most frequently in the head and neck. It usually occurs within the first week to 3 months after

| Table 2<br>First-generation or conventional antipsychotics | | |
| --- | --- | --- |
| **High Potency** | **Medium Potency** | **Low Potency** |
| Haloperidol (Haldol)<br>Fluphenazine (Prolixin)<br>Thiothixene (Navane)<br>Trifluoperazine (Stelazine) | Loxipine (Loxitane)—acts as an<br>    atypical at low doses<br>Perphenazine (Trilafon) | Chlorpromazine (Thorazine)<br>Thioridazine (Mellaril) |

antipsychotic initiation. Management includes intramuscular diphenhydramine or benztropine, a short course of an oral anticholinergic (prevent recurrence), slower dose titration, or switch to a different antipsychotic.

Tardive dyskinesia: involuntary movements of the face and mouth (blinking, lip smacking, or writhing movements of the neck, back, trunk, and/or limbs). It occurs after long-term antipsychotic administration and may not be reversible, even if an agent is discontinued. Management includes discontinuing the antipsychotic or switching to lower-risk agent (clozapine), if possible.

Drug-induced parkinsonisms: resting hand tremors, decreased movement (mask-like facies, bradykinesia, loss of facial expression, and flattening of vocal inflection), stiffness (cogwheel and lead pipe rigidity), drooling, and shuffling gait. Management includes reducing antipsychotic dose, changing the agent, and using an oral antiparkinson or anticholinergic agent. Pharmacologic treatment should be tapered to discontinuation every 4 to 6 weeks to reassess symptoms.

*Hyperprolactinemia*

Blockade of $D_2$ in the tuberoinfundibular pathway by antipsychotics may lead to hyperprolactinemia. Elevated prolactin can cause galactorrhea, amenorrhea, or gynecomastia. Studies have found a correlation between chronic hyperprolactinemia and osteoporosis.[10] The agents most commonly implicated in hyperprolactinemia are high-potency FGAs, risperidone, paliperidone, and low-potency FGAs. Prolactin levels are not routinely drawn but can be checked if symptoms occur. Interventions include monitoring patients for symptoms of hyperprolactinemia, checking prolactin levels when symptomatic, and switching to an agent with less potential for hyperprolactinemia like aripiprazole or quetiapine.[7]

### Second-generation (or Atypical) Antipsychotics

Like FGAs, SGAs block $D_2$ receptors, but they also exhibit activity at serotonin receptors. Activity at $D_2$ and serotonin receptors allows SGAs to treat psychosis while having lower risk for extrapyramidal symptoms and hyperprolactinemia. The major concerns with SGAs are metabolic changes. Weight gain may occur independent of dose.[7] Aside from weight gain, SGAs may cause hyperglycemia and dyslipidemia. Clozapine and olanzapine carry the highest risk of metabolic consequences. Quetiapine has an intermediate risk for metabolic changes, and the remaining SGAs are associated with a low risk. During treatment with SGAs, metabolic parameters, such as weight, body mass index, hemoglobin $A_{1c}$, and lipids should be routinely monitored. Lifestyle changes, such as eating a healthy diet and incorporating moderate exercise, should be encouraged at the time of prescribing to prevent weight gain.[11,12]

Clozapine has been shown more effective than other antipsychotics agents in managing patients with treatment-resistant schizophrenia and suicidality.[13] Clozapine does not cause movement abnormalities but is associated with a hematologic ADR and agranulocytosis. Agranulocytosis occurs in 1% to 2% of patients taking clozapine. Guidelines exist to dictate the frequency of complete blood cell count (CBC) monitoring and actions to take should CBC changes occur. Patients and providers must be enrolled in a national registry and CBC information must be entered to prescribe clozapine. Additional SEs and ADRs of clozapine include seizures, myocarditis, sialorrhea, and constipation. Nurses can have an impact on clozapine therapy by ensuring dosing guidelines are followed to prevent ADRs and educating patients on signs and symptoms of agranulocytosis (mouth sores, fever, sore throat, and weakness) and myocarditis (fatigue, dyspnea, chest pain, and fever). Interventions for sialorrhea include sugarless chewing gum, elevating the head while sleeping, and keeping a towel or napkin available. Increasing fiber intake, hydration, and physical activity can help with constipation.

## Adverse Drug Reactions and Side Effects that May Occur with First-generation Antipsychotics and Second-generation Antipsychotics

### Neuroleptic malignant syndrome

The exact pathophysiology of neuroleptic malignant syndrome (NMS) is not fully understood but is thought to occur after abrupt and drastic reduction in $D_2$ by medications affecting the central dopaminergic system.[14] Although antipsychotics are most commonly implicated, $D_2$-altering agents, such as metoclopramide, amoxapine, lithium, and phenelzine, also have been reported to cause NMS. Studies suggest 0.01% to 0.02% of patients exposed to antipsychotics develop NMS.[15] The incidence of NMS is low, but health care providers must be vigilant because the estimated mortality rate is 10%.[16]

Accurately diagnosing NMS is crucial because this condition can be life threatening and requires immediate treatment. The diagnosed is based on laboratory studies, vital signs, physical and mental status examination, history of exposure to $D_2$ blocking agent, and the presence of clinical signs and symptoms (**Table 3**). NMS may occur after days or months of antipsychotic administration. A patient's physical history may reveal additional risk factors associated with NMS, such as dehydration, physical exhaustion, parenteral administration of $D_2$ blocking agents, polypharmacy, rapid titration, or high dose.[14] Treatment involves supportive measures to stabilize cardiovascular function, reduce body temperature, promote oxygenation, and reduce rigidity. There is much controversy regarding the utility of pharmacotherapy in NMS. Agents that have been used include dantrolene and bromocriptine. If dantrolene is chosen, liver function tests should be monitored to assess for dantrolene-induced hepatitis.[17] Additional nursing interventions include monitoring mental and physical status during NMS treatment.

### Corrected QT prolongation

Antipsychotics can prolong the corrected QT (QTc) interval, which may lead to an arrhythmia known as torsade de pointes. Normal QTc levels are less than 450 ms for men and 470 ms for women. A threshold for clinical concern has not been firmly established, but clinical evaluation and consideration of drug discontinuation should occur when QTc exceeds 500 ms or increases 20 ms to 60 ms or more from baseline.[18]

The risk of QTc prolongation and torsade de pointes varies by agent and depends on several factors. Thioridazine has the highest documented risk and lurasidone has the lowest risk.[19] Risk factors for QTc prolongation include age greater than 65, higher doses, interacting medications, use of multiple QTc-prolonging medications, congenital long QT syndrome, family history of sudden death, personal history of cardiac disease, and electrolyte disturbances. Care should be taken to avoid using

| Table 3 | | | |
|---|---|---|---|
| **Manifestations of neuroleptic malignant syndrome** | | | |
| Severe Muscle Rigidity | Diaphoresis | Tremor | High or Labile Blood Pressure |
| Fever | Hypoxia | Altered mental status | Creatine kinase elevation |
| Tachycardia | Incontinence | Dysphagia | Leukocytosis |

antipsychotics in combination with other medications that prolong the QTc interval, such as class I and III antiarrhythmic agents, TCAs, and some antibiotics, to name a few. There are several other agents with the potential to prolong the QTc interval. The Web site, crediblemeds.org, is a good resource to check a medication's cardiac risk. Nursing interventions include

- Monitoring electrolytes and correcting abnormalities, especially hypomagnesemia, hypocalcemia, and hypokalemia
- Recommending ECG monitoring for patients with
  - Pulse less than 50 beats per minute
  - Low potassium, calcium, or magnesium
  - Family history of congenital long QT syndrome
  - Suspected medication overdose
  - Risk factors for QTc prolongation and/or prescription of a high-risk agent
  - Unexplained cardiac arrest, loss of consciousness, or syncope

## LONG-ACTING INJECTABLE ANTIPSYCHOTICS

Several antipsychotics are available as long-acting injections (**Box 2**). The benefit of these agents is less frequent dosing and improved compliance in patients unable to take medications daily. As a general rule, tolerance should be established with a trial of the oral agent prior to administering the long-acting injection. For patients who receive paliperidone palmitate, risperidone or paliperidone may be used for the oral trial, because paliperidone is a metabolite of risperidone. SEs of long-acting injectable antipsychotics are generally similar to the parent compound with the addition of injection site reactions (**Table 4**).[20] Olanzapine pamoate injection carries a black box warning for postinjection sedation and delirium. Patients can only receive olanzapine pamoate injections by trained professionals in a health care facility with access to an emergency department, and patients must be monitored for at least 3 hours after the injection.

| Table 4 Interventions for common side effects associated with antipsychotics | |
| --- | --- |
| **Side Effect** | **Intervention** |
| Sedation | Reduce the dose, consolidate administration to a single bedtime dose, or switch to a less sedating agent |
| Dry mouth | Sugarless gum or candy or provide oral hygiene |
| Orthostatic hypotension | Counsel patient to rise slowly from lying or sitting positions, monitor blood pressure, increase fluid intake if not contraindicated, reduce the dose, switch to a different agent |
| Weight gain | Eat a balanced diet, exercise regularly |

## ANTIDEPRESSANTS

Depression places a significant burden on patients, families, communities, and the health care system. The first selective serotonin reuptake inhibitor (SSRI), fluoxetine (Prozac), entered the market in 1987. Since then, additional SSRIs and conventional antidepressants have been discovered. Although SSRIs are the most commonly prescribed antidepressant medications, serotonin-norepinephrine reuptake inhibitors (SNRIs), bupropion, and other agents are also commonly used (**Box 3**).

---

**Box 2**
**Available long-acting injectable antipsychotics**

Fluphenazine decanoate (Prolixin Decanoate)

Risperidone long-acting injection (Risperdal Consta)

Olanzapine pamoate (Zyprexa Relprevv)

Haloperidol decanoate (Haldol Decanoate)

Paliperidone palmitate (Invega Sustenna and Invega Trinza)

Aripiprazole extended-release injection (Abilify Maintena)

---

### Selective Serotonin Reuptake Inhibitors

Common SEs of SSRIs include gastrointestinal (GI) disturbances, weight changes, sleep disturbance, anxiety, tremor, akathisia, headache, and sexual dysfunction. GI SEs, such as anorexia, nausea, and diarrhea, are usually transient and resolve over the course of therapy. There is a higher incidence of GI upset with sertraline. SSRIs may also cause activating SEs (insomnia, anxiety, and tremor) in the first 1 to 2 weeks of treatment. Fluoxetine is the most activating SSRI and paroxetine is the most sedating. SSRIs can cause sexual dysfunction, which is bothersome for patients and may lead to noncompliance. When sexual SEs occur, interventions include lowering the dose or switching to an agent with fewer sexual SEs, such as bupropion.[21] SSRIs may rarely cause hyponatremia. Older adults and patients and patients taking diuretics have a greater risk of SSRI-induced hyponatremia. Electrolytes should be monitored at baseline and as clinically indicated. If a patient develops symptomatic hyponatremia, the agent should be discontinued and the patient should receive appropriate treatment of hyponatremia.

### Other Antidepressants

The SNRIs, venlafaxine (Effexor), desvenlafaxine (Pristiq), duloxetine (Cymbalta), and levomilnacipran (Fetzima), represent another popular class of antidepressants. SNRIs may cause elevations in blood pressure and heart rate; therefore, vital signs should be routinely monitored during SNRI therapy.[22,23] Class SEs include dizziness, headache, sleep disturbances, sexual dysfunction, and GI upset. At low doses, venlafaxine behaves as an SSRI.

Vilazodone (Viibryd) is a serotonin partial agonist and reuptake inhibitor. SEs include GI upset and sleep disturbances. Vortioxetine (Brintellix) is a novel serotonin modulator.[24] The most commonly occurring SEs with vortioxetine are nausea, diarrhea,

---

**Box 3**
**Selective serotonin reuptake inhibitors**

Fluoxetine (Prozac)

Sertraline (Zoloft)

Paroxetine (Paxil)

Escitalopram (Lexapro)

Citalopram (Celexa)

---

constipation, vomiting, and dizziness. Headaches, sexual dysfunction, and nasopharyngitis have also been reported with vortioxetine.

Trazodone (Desyrel) and nefazodone (Serzone) are serotonin antagonist/reuptake inhibitors. They share similar SE profiles, including sedation, dry mouth, dizziness, orthostatic hypotension, and blurred vision.[22] Trazodone carries a risk of priapism. Patients should be counseled to seek immediate medical attention for an erection that is painful or lasts longer than 4 hours. Nefazodone is used less commonly due to the risk of elevated liver enzymes. Patients should be counseled to report signs of hepatitis, such as yellowing of the skin or eyes, weakness, abdominal pain, lethargy, and clay-colored stools.

Bupropion (Wellbutrin) is a norepinephrine-$D_2$ reuptake inhibitor with stimulating properties. ADRs associated with bupropion include agitation, dry mouth, headache, tremor, and insomnia.[22] A more serious consequence of stimulation during bupropion therapy is seizure. Patients with a history of seizures should avoid bupropion use. To reduce the risk of seizures in patients taking bupropion, the dose should be slowly titrated and should not exceeded recommended doses, which depend on product formulation.

Mirtazapine (Remeron) is a presynaptic $\alpha_2$-antagonist. SEs of mirtazapine include sedation, dry mouth, increased appetite, weight gain, and hypertriglyceridemia. Mirtazapine is more sedating at low doses compared with higher doses. Weight and triglycerides should be monitored during mirtazapine therapy (**Table 5**).

### Serotonin Syndrome

Serotonin syndrome is an ADR caused by overactivation of central and peripheral serotonin receptors after the use of serotonergic medications. Serotonin syndrome may be precipitated by use of a single serotonergic drug, an overdose involving a serotonergic drug, or concomitant use of 2 or more serotonergic agents.[25] Serotonin-altering medications include antidepressants, such as MAOIs, TCAs, SSRIs, SNRIs, mirtazapine, and trazodone. Other medications, such as tramadol, linezolid, meperidine, dextromethorphan, and the herbal St. John's wort, have also been implicated in cases of serotonin syndrome. Prevention is the major nursing intervention. All patients prescribed serotonergic psychotropics should be counseled on medications that precipitate serotonin syndrome as well as the signs and symptoms of this ADR (**Table 6**).

| Table 5 | |
|---|---|
| **Common antidepressant side effects and management** | |
| **Side Effect** | **Management** |
| GI disturbances | Counsel that symptoms usually resolve over time, take medication with food, lower the dose, take at bedtime, or change agent |
| Weight gain | Consume a balanced diet, exercise regularly |
| Tremor, akathisia, anxiety | Slowly titrate the dose, maintain on the lowest effect dose, educate the patient to report movement abnormalities, anxiety, restlessness, or agitation |
| Sleep disturbances | For insomnia: move dose to morning, ensure second dose is taken in early evening (if dosed multiple times per day) For sedation: switch dosing to bedtime |
| Headaches | Reduce the dose, take medication at bedtime, switch antidepressant, educate the patient on relaxation techniques, offer nonnarcotic analgesics, such as ibuprofen and acetaminophen, if not contraindicated |

| Table 6 Symptoms of serotonin syndrome | | |
|---|---|---|
| Mental Status Changes | Hyperthermia | Hyperreflexia |
| Labile blood pressure and pulse | Elevated creatine kinase | Myoclonus |
| Tremor | Vomiting/diarrhea | Diaphoresis |
| Muscle rigidity | Mydriasis | Flushed skin |

Treatment includes discontinuing serotonergic medications, providing supportive care, and sedation with benzodiazepines in cases of agitation.[25] Serotonin antagonists, such as cyproheptadine, may be administered for autonomic instability.

### Suicide Risk and Mania

All antidepressants carry a black box warning for increased risk of suicidal thoughts and behaviors in children, adolescents, and young adults 18 to 24 years of age. Suicide risk should be closely monitored in patients prescribed antidepressants.[26] Additionally, patients should be monitored for mania and hypomania when initiating antidepressants. Mania may occur when antidepressants are started, especially in patients with undiagnosed bipolar disorder. If mania occurs, the antidepressant should be discontinued pending further evaluation. If a patient is found to have bipolar disorder, the goal of treatment should change to mood stabilization.[27]

### Withdrawal

Withdrawal symptoms may occur with abrupt discontinuation of SSRIs and many newer antidepressant agents. Symptoms of withdrawal can range in severity and include dizziness, paresthesias, flulike symptoms, nausea, myalgias, insomnia, anxiety, and irritability.[28] Withdrawal occurs most frequently with paroxetine and venlafaxine (due to short half-life) and less commonly with fluoxetine (due to long half-life). To prevent withdrawal symptoms, patients should be encouraged to take their medications every day. Patients should not stop taking antidepressants without consulting their medical provider. Tapering must be done slowly. If withdrawal symptoms occur during the course of tapering, the dose should be raised to the last tolerated dose and tapering should resume at a slower rate.

## MOOD STABILIZERS

Lithium and antiepileptic medications, such as valproic acid (VPA), carbamazepine (CBZ), and lamotrigine, are often used as mood stabilizers in the treatment of bipolar disorder. Atypical antipsychotics may also be used; however, these agents were previously discussed. Nonadherence to mood stabilizers ranges from 10% to 60% in bipolar disorder and can often be attributed to SEs.[3] Common SEs encountered with mood stabilizers include weight gain (except with lamotrigine, which is weight neutral), sedation, sexual dysfunction, alopecia, and cognitive deficits. All mood stabilizers are teratogenic and this fact must be discussed with women of childbearing potential. Nursing interventions for SEs are crucial for improving patient safety and compliance with mood stabilizers.

### Lithium

Common SEs of lithium include weight gain (dose and duration dependent), GI upset, hand tremor, and cognitive effects. Patients on lithium may also develop polydipsia, polyuria, diabetes insipidus, leukocytosis, ECG changes, or hypothyroidism.[3,29] Baseline laboratory and cardiac studies should be performed prior to starting lithium and routinely as indicated. Patients should be educated to drink adequate fluid to avoid dehydration. Diabetes insipidus can be treated with diuretics. Lithium-induced leukocytosis is usually benign and does not require medication discontinuation. If symptomatic, hypothyroidism may be treated with thyroid supplement and lithium can be continued. Lithium has a narrow therapeutic window; therefore, a major nursing intervention includes monitoring serum lithium levels. The therapeutic lithium range is 0.6 mEq/L to 1.5 mEq/L. Lithium toxicity may occur at any lithium level, but toxic symptoms often correlate with serum level. If lithium toxicity is suspected, the mood stabilizer should be discontinued. Dehydration, decrease in salt intake, sweating, diuretics, angiotensin-converting enzyme inhibitors, and diarrhea increase the risk of lithium toxicity (**Table 7**).

### Divalproex Sodium or Valproic Acid

Common SEs of VPA are weight gain, GI upset, sedation, and tremor. VPA may also cause hepatitis, pancreatitis, hematologic abnormalities, and hyperammonemia.[3,29] Patients taking VPA should be educated on the signs and symptoms of pancreatitis and hepatitis. VPA should be used with caution in patients with a history of liver disease and should be discontinued if liver function tests exceed 2 to 3 times the upper limit of normal. CBC should be evaluated at baseline and as clinically indicated to assess for hematologic changes, such as thrombocytopenia or leukopenia. Ammonia levels should be checked if sudden mental status changes occur. Hyperammonemia can be treated with a short course of lactulose. Liver function should be checked at baseline and routinely during treatment. Similar to lithium, VPA has a narrow therapeutic index and levels should be monitored. The therapeutic range in bipolar disorder is 50 μg/mL to 125 μg/mL.

### Carbamazepine

CBZ is another anticonvulsant used for mood stabilization. Common SEs of CBZ include sedation, dizziness, anticholinergic effects, diplopia, and transient liver function test elevations. If diplopia occurs, a different agent should be chosen. More concerning ADRs with CBZ include hematologic changes, such as aplastic anemia and leukopenia, Stevens-Johnson syndrome (SJS), and hyponatremia.[3,29] CBC should be monitored, and patients should be educated to report symptoms of agranulocytosis and any rashes. The rash, SJS, is most common in patients with the HLA-B*1502 allele, which is found mostly in people of Chinese descent. Genetic testing can screen for this allele. Patients with the HLA-B*1502 allele should not take CBZ.

| Table 7 Lithium toxicity and possible symptoms | | |
|---|---|---|
| **Severity of Toxicity** | **Level** | **Symptoms** |
| Mild toxicity | 1.5–2.0 mEq/L | GI upset, lethargy, tremor, weakness |
| Moderate toxicity | 2.0–2.5 mEq/L | Severe GI upset, confusion, nystagmus, ataxia |
| Severe toxicity | >2.5 mEq/L | Severe GI upset, impaired consciousness, seizures, syncope, coma |

| Table 8 Interventions for mood stabilizer–induced side effects | |
|---|---|
| Sedation | Switch Dosing to Bedtime |
| Tremor | Switch to extended-release formulations, reducing caffeine or nicotine consumption may be helpful, treat tremor with propranolol, minimize polypharmacy if possible |
| GI SEs | Switch to enteric-coated or controlled-release products; take medication with food; consider bedtime dosing, dose reduction, or gradual dose titration; educate patients GI upset is usually transient |
| Weight gain | Consume a balanced diet, exercise regularly, switch agent |
| Alopecia | Slow dose titration, selenium and zinc supplementation, hair replacement |

Plasma levels can be monitored with CBZ and should be maintained at 8 μg/mL to 12 μg/mL.

### Lamotrigine

Lamotrigine has also been associated with the development of SJS or toxic necrolysis.[3,29] Lamotrigine dose is titrated over several weeks to avoid rashes. If a patient stops lamotrigine, the dose titration must start over. If a rash develops, lamotrigine should be discontinued. The rash should be treated appropriately, and lamotrigine should not be reinitiated unless it is determined the rash was not drug related (**Table 8**).

### STIMULANTS

Stimulant medications, such as methylphenidate and amphetamines, are approved for initial treatment of attention-deficit/hyperactivity disorder. These medications work by inhibiting reuptake or stimulating release of $D_2$ and norepinephrine. Common SEs of stimulants include decreased appetite, insomnia, GI upset, headache, and skin irritation with transdermal patch.[30] Management for common stimulant SEs is discussed in **Table 9**. Stimulants may also raise blood pressure and carry a black box warning for risk of abuse and dependence. Patients should be closely monitored for signs of abuse and vital signs should be monitored while taking stimulants. Use of stimulants is not recommended in patients with arteriosclerosis, symptomatic cardiovascular diseases, moderate to severe hypertension, hyperthyroidism, and history of drug abuse. Stimulants should not be administered within 14 days of MAOI use. Due to $D_2$-enhancing effects, patients should be monitored for stimulant-induced psychosis or mania.

| Table 9 Stimulant side effects and management | |
|---|---|
| Decreased appetite | Eat balanced meals, monitor weight, switch to nonstimulant medication |
| Insomnia | Change to short-acting agent, reduce afternoon doses or take earlier in the day |
| GI upset | Take with food |
| Headache | Lower or divide dose, non-narcotic analgesics |
| Skin irritation | Rotate patch application site |

## SUMMARY

Over the years, newer psychotropic agents have been developed with the goal of minimizing risks and optimizing therapeutic benefits. To date, there is no perfect medication to treat mental illnesses; therefore, health care providers must be aware of SEs and ADRs as well as applicable management. Nursing interventions that focus on early identification, prevention, and appropriate management of ADRs can greatly improve health care for patients receiving psychotropic medications.

## REFERENCES

1. WHO. Handbook of Resolutions and Decisions of the World Health Assembly and Executive Board. In: WHA 16.36 Clinical and pharmacological evaluation of drugs. Geneva (Switzerland): WHO; 1973. p. 1948–72.
2. Edwards I, Aronson J. Adverse drug reactions: definitions, diagnosis, and management. Lancet 2000;356(9237):1255–9.
3. Dols A, Sienaert P, Van gerven H, et al. The prevalence and management of side effects of lithium and anticonvulsants as mood stabilizers in bipolar disorder from a clinical perspective: a review. Int Clin Psychopharmacol 2013;28(6):287–96.
4. Jemal A, Ward E, Hao Y, et al. Trends in the leading causes of death in the United States in years 1970–2002. JAMA 2005;294:1255–9.
5. Alomar MJ. Factors affecting the development of adverse drug reactions (Review article). Saudi Pharm J 2014;22(2):83–94.
6. Dibonaventura M, Gabriel S, Dupclay L, et al. A patient perspective of the impact of medication side effects on adherence: results of a cross-sectional nationwide survey of patients with schizophrenia. BMC Psychiatry 2012;12(1):20.
7. Muench J, Hamer AM. Adverse effects of antipsychotic medications. Am Fam Physician 2010;81(5):617–22.
8. Hieber R. Movement disorder toolbox [Internet]. Ment Health Clin 2012;1(7): 153–5.
9. Mehta SH, Morgan JC, Sethi KD. Drug-induced movement disorders. Neurol Clin 2015;33(1):153–74.
10. Howard L, Kirkwood G, Leese M. Risk of hip fracture in patients with a history of schizophrenia. Br J Psychiatry 2007;190:129–34.
11. Domecq JP, Prutsky G, Leppin A, et al. Clinical review: drugs commonly associated with weight change: a systematic review and meta-analysis. J Clin Endocrinol Metab 2015;100(2):363–70.
12. Green CA, Yarborough BJ, Leo MC, et al. The STRIDE weight loss and lifestyle intervention for individuals taking antipsychotic medications: a randomized trial. Am J Psychiatry 2015;172(1):71–81.
13. Sagy R, Weizman A, Katz N. Pharmacological and behavioral management of some often-overlooked clozapine-induced side effects. Int Clin Psychopharmacol 2014;29(6):313–7.
14. Langan J, Martin D, Shajahan P, et al. Antipsychotic dose escalation as a trigger for neuroleptic malignant syndrome (NMS): literature review and case series report. BMC Psychiatry 2012;12:214.
15. Spivak B, Maline DI, Kozyrev VN, et al. Frequency of neuroleptic malignant syndrome in a large psychiatric hospital in Moscow. Eur Psychiatry 2000;15(5): 330–3.
16. Strawn JR, Keck PE, Caroff SN. Neuroleptic malignant syndrome. Am J Psychiatry 2007;164(6):870–6.

17. Pelonero AL, Levenson JL, Pandurangi AK. Neuroleptic malignant syndrome: a review. Psychiatr Serv 1998;49(9):1163–72.
18. Haverkamp W, Breithardt G, Camm AJ, et al. The potential for QT prolongation and pro-arrhythmia by non-antiarrhythmic drugs: clinical and regulatory implications. Report on a Policy Conference of the European Society of Cardiology. Cardiovasc Res 2000;47:219–33.
19. Shah AA, Aftab A, Coverdale J. QTc prolongation with antipsychotics: is routine ECG monitoring recommended? J Psychiatr Pract 2014;20(3):196–206.
20. Gentile S. Adverse effects associated with second-generation antipsychotic long-acting injection treatment: a comprehensive systematic review. Pharmacotherapy 2013;33(10):1087–106.
21. Montejo AL, Montejo L, Navarro-cremades F. Sexual side-effects of antidepressant and antipsychotic drugs. Curr Opin Psychiatry 2015;28(6):418–23.
22. Papakostas GI. Tolerability of modern antidepressants. J Clin Psychiatry 2008; 69(Suppl E1):8–13.
23. Forest Pharamceuticals Inc. FetzimaTM (levomilnacipran) extended-release capsules, for oral use: US prescribing information. 2013. Available at: http://www.frx.com/pi/fetzima_pi.pdf. Accessed September 01, 2015.
24. Takeda Pharmaceuticals America, Inc. Brintellix (vortioxetine) tablets, for oral use. 2013. Available at: http://www.accessdata.fda.gov/drugsatfda_docs/label/2013/204447s000lbl.pdf. Accessed October 15, 2015.
25. Volpi-abadie J, Kaye AM, Kaye AD. Serotonin syndrome. Ochsner J 2013;13(4): 533–40.
26. Isacsson G, Rich CL. Antidepressant drugs and the risk of suicide in children and adolescents. Paediatr Drugs 2014;16(2):115–22.
27. Viktorin A, Lichtenstein P, Thase ME, et al. The risk of switch to mania in patients with bipolar disorder during treatment with an antidepressant alone and in combination with a mood stabilizer. Am J Psychiatry 2014;171(10):1067–73.
28. Ogle NR, Akkerman SR. Guidance for the discontinuation or switching of antidepressant therapies in adults. J Pharm Pract 2013;26(4):389–96.
29. Kemp DE. Managing the side effects associated with commonly used treatments for bipolar depression. J Affect Disord 2014;169(Suppl 1):S34–44.
30. Santosh PJ, Sattar S, Canagaratnam M. Efficacy and tolerability of pharmacotherapies for attention-deficit hyperactivity disorder in adults. CNS Drugs 2011;25(9): 737–63.

# Caring for Trauma Survivors

Deborah Antai-Otong, MS, APRN, PMHCNS-BC, FAAN

## KEYWORDS

- Trauma • Trauma-informed care • Posttraumatic stress disorder • Vicarious trauma
- Dissociation • Resilience • Self-care

## KEY POINTS

- Define trauma and contributing factors associated with its aftermath.
- Review major concepts of trauma-informed care.
- Review the role of the psychiatric nurse in caring for trauma survivors.
- Describe evidence-based pharmacologic and psychotherapeutic approaches used in the treatment of trauma and stress-related disorders.

## INTRODUCTION

Trauma results from an overwhelming encounter with an intense or distressful experience, such as rape or witnessing a murder, that causes emotional and psychological stress reactions. Trauma can and does impact the lives of all cultures, races, ethnicities, gender, ages, communities, and countries. Symptoms of trauma stem from the individual's adaptation to the traumatic event. Traumatic experiences are capable of producing adverse acute and long-term consequences. Typically, acute stress reactions emerge immediately after an exposure to a trauma and may manifest as intense anxiety and fearfulness, and concentration and sleep disturbances.[1] Researchers submit that the long-term impact of trauma exposure is linked to a myriad of mental health and physical disorders that contribute to the high use of primary care and emergency department resources by trauma survivors.[2]

## PREVALENCE

Sixty percent of people encounter at least 1 traumatic event in their lives, but only a small percentage develop posttraumatic stress disorders (PTSD) or other psychiatric disorders.[3] Findings from the National Comorbidity study indicate that only 7% of people exposed to traumatic events will develop PTSD.[4] These data further indicate that approximately 20% of women and 8% of men will develop PTSD. Bryant and

Disclosure: None.
Department of Veterans Affairs, Veterans Integrated Service Networks-(VISN-17), 2301 E. Lamar Boulevard, Arlington, TX 76006, USA
E-mail address: Deborah.Antai-Otong@va.gov

colleagues[5] assert that trauma reactions vary among people and that complete recovery occurs within 3 months in about 50% of trauma surveyors. In comparison, others may experience trauma reactions for 12 months or longer.[5] A considerable body of research purports that trauma survivors who develop stress-related disorders, such as PTSD, experience persistent exaggerated stress responses.

PTSD is the most commonly recognized psychiatric disorder after a traumatic event.[3,4] This quintessential and disabling psychiatric disorder frequently cooccurs with 1 or more psychiatric and physical disorders.[4] Common cooccurring psychiatric disorders associated with PTSD include depression, substance use disorders, and borderline personality disorders, all of which increase the risk of suicide.[6] Major physical problems linked to chronic stress disorders include cardiovascular disease and autoimmune disorders (ie, fibromyalgia, multiple sclerosis).[7–9] Trauma survivors are also likely to report an increased suicide or self-harm risk, impaired employment and interpersonal relationships, and poor quality of life.[10] Many trauma survivors seek services in primary care settings and present with unique health care needs.[2]

Considering the emerging number of individuals exposed to trauma, psychiatric nurses need to be knowledgeable of trauma and stress-related disorders and early interventions that mitigate their long-term adverse outcomes, particularly in vulnerable populations. Vulnerable populations include those who are younger, females, and combat soldiers. Equally important is for psychiatric nurses to recognize signs and symptoms of acute and chronic stress reactions and initiate nursing interventions that are strength based and person centric, and facilitate an optimal level of functioning and recovery.

This paper discusses the role of psychiatric mental health nurses in the identification, assessment, and treatment of patients who survive acute and chronic trauma. Core competencies associated with helping trauma survivors recover begin with understanding major underpinnings and core features of trauma reactions, establishing nurse–patient relationships guided by trauma-informed care, implementing trauma-specific care, and establishing collaborative relationships.

## CAUSES OF TRAUMA AND STRESS-RELATED DISORDERS

The precise cause of trauma and stress-related disorders remains obscure, but most studies indicate that they arise from persistent or dysregulation of stress responses that are mediated by complex and multifaceted underpinnings.[11] A discussion of the multifaceted and complexity of trauma and stress-related disorders is beyond the scope of this article. However, it is well-documented that major determinants of the development of PTSD are vast. Major determinants include the type and severity of trauma exposure, ability to modulate emotional responsiveness, coexisting psychiatric disorders, personality and genetic factors, and quality of adaptive coping or resilience and problem-solving skills.[12–15] These factors are believed to mediate how one perceives the threat, modulates stress responses, mobilizes adaptive coping skills, and recovers from the event.

Consistent research implicates various neural pathways in stress modulation and memory formation after a traumatic event. For example, the nucleus incertus-hippocampus and medial prefrontal cortical pathway is implicated in stress responses and believed to play a dominant role in maladaptive stress responses.[14–16]

Supposedly, traumatic events activate the nucleus incertus via the corticotropin-releasing factor type 1 receptor stimulation suppresses the hippocampal–medial prefrontal cortical–key neural processes associated with the ability to mitigate or dampen stress responses.[15,16] Chronic stress responses cause dysregulation of the medial prefrontal cortical, which subsequently impairs working memory and fear memory consolidation (permanent memory formation) and other cognitive responses related to accurate recalls of the traumatic event.[15–17] (see Deborah Antai-Otong: Anxiety Disorders: Treatment Considerations, in this issue for a more detailed discussion of causative factors and underpinnings associated with trauma and stress-related disorders [ie, PTSD]).

The following section focuses on core features of trauma and stress-related disorders.

## CORE FEATURES OF TRAUMA AND STRESS-RELATED DISORDERS

In 2013, the American Psychiatric Association[1] published the fifth edition of the Diagnostic Statistical Manual of Mental Disorders (DSM-V). The DSM-V created a distinct cluster of psychiatric disorders that more accurately reflects trauma and stress-related disorders more than the cluster of anxiety disorders. In order for a person to be diagnosed with PTSD and stress-related disorders it is necessary meet the first criterion of being exposed to a devastating and intense trauma either directly, witnessing an event that affects others, learning of a traumatic event that effects a significant other, or experiencing recurrent or extreme exposure to aversive aspects of a traumatic event. Additional criteria include stress-related behavioral symptoms, specifically reexperiencing, avoidance, negative cognitions and mood, and arousal.[1]

Reexperiencing entails unprompted recurrent memories or images of the traumatic event (ie, nightmares, dissociative flashbacks). Dissociative states are related to disturbances in memory, personal identity, and perceptions. Studies indicate that dissociation is a predictor of long-term adverse outcomes of trauma exposure, such as PTSD.[18] Avoidance behaviors refer to dampening or avoiding feelings, thoughts, people, places, and events that trigger memories of the traumatic event. Symptoms of arousal include irritability, anger, hypervigilance, exaggerated startle reactions, and reduced concentration and sleep disturbances. Negative cognitions and mood refer to recurring and exaggerated negative thoughts, beliefs about self, others, and the world, a sense of self-blame, and an inability to experience positive experiences.[1]

For the purpose of this article, the discussion of these diagnostic categories will be limited to acute stress disorder and PTSD. Acute stress disorder is described as an immediate stress reaction that occurs within 3 days to 1 month of exposure to an overwhelming traumatic event. According to researchers, the frequency in which acute stress disorder develops in trauma survivors is determined by the nature of the event and the environment in which it is assessed. Acute stress disorder symptoms are distinguished from PTSD because the duration of symptoms are restricted to a duration of 3 days and up to 1 month compared with PTSD symptoms, which endure a month or longer. Recent accounts of the rationale for the diagnostic category of acute stress disorder in the DSM-V criteria[1] is related to the identification of these patients seem to have a higher propensity to develop PTSD or future psychiatric disorders. Furthermore, it is useful in assessing high-risk populations and affording early interventions to trauma survivors during the immediate period after a traumatic event.[19]

## TRAUMA-INFORMED CARE

Trauma-informed care is an evidence-based approach that psychiatric nurses can use to facilitate positive adaptive coping and problem solving skills, recovery, and resilience.[20] The Consensus-based definition of trauma-informed care is:

*a strengths-based framework that is grounded in an understanding of and responsiveness to the impact of trauma, that emphasizes physical, psychological, and emotional safety for both providers and survivors, and that creates opportunities for survivors to rebuild a sense of control and empowerment.*[20(p82)]

Guiding principles trauma-informed care are to address the needs of trauma survivors while providing immediate emotional support. Successful implementation of trauma-informed care involves a philosophic paradigm shift that integrates a system-wide responsiveness and understanding of trauma. This transformation requires cultural changes in mental health and primary care settings that begin with the initial contact with the patient. For the purpose of this paper, the implementation of these principles are limited to the nurse-patient encounters. Trauma-informed care also requires psychiatric nurses to establish healing relationships that address the aftermath of trauma or trauma awareness, emphasize safety, provide opportunities to reclaim control, and be person centered and strength based[20–22] **(Box 1)**.

## TRAUMA SCREENING AND ASSESSMENT

It is important to approach the patient with sincere respect, concern, and knowledge of normal and trauma-related stress reactions. Engaging the patient in a therapeutic

---

**Box 1**
**Trauma screening**

- Use nonthreatening body language.
- Anticipate various environmental cues that may cause intense emotional reactions, such as access to exit, seating, loud noises, or raised voice.
- Discuss rationale for trauma screening and explain what to expect during the assessment and screening process.
- Tailor tone of voice, volume, and rate to the patient's emotional state.
- Avoid rushing or frequently looking at time.
- Ensure ample space and avoid invading the survivor's personal space.
- Be cognizant and sensitive to cultural symbols associated with a safe environment.
- Follow the survivor's lead and assess emotional and physiologic responses to questions.
- Exhibit clear message about your availability and accessibility throughout the assessment and treatment.
- It may be less threatening to assess a broad perspective of current and historical experiences.
- Use clear, behaviorally based questions.
- Avoid behaviors or experiences that may result in retraumatization such as:
  - Not allowing involvement in treatment decisions;
  - Mislabeling behaviors as "personality disorder" or mental health; and
  - Problem versus traumatic stress reaction.
- Foster control, preferences, and independence.
- Take "small steps" in history gathering.
- Educate about potential consequences trauma and available resources and referrals.
- Collaborate with mental health professionals.
- Establish and maintain therapeutic boundaries.
- Be aware of your own reactions to the survivor's trauma history, particularly in the face of intense and challenging survivor reactions.[20–22,27]

*Data from* Refs.[20–22,28]

relationship promotes trust and acceptance. Trauma survivors often struggle with sharing an accurate account of the trauma and may also be hesitant to share details because they feel ashamed and fear they will be retraumatized. It is important for the nurse to answer questions about what the patient may be experiencing; normalize stress reactions; build resilience; educate about effective coping skills, while respecting the patient's individual coping choices; and most important provide a positive experience. A positive experience increases the chances of the patient seeking future help if needed. It also enables the nurse to explore the meaning of the patient's traumatic experience and assess trauma-related stress reactions.[21]

During these seemingly overwhelming and intense nurse–patient interactions, it is imperative for nurses to monitor their personal feelings, thoughts, and behavioral and biologic reactions to the patient's experience. Self-awareness is the foundation of empathy. Through empathy, the nurse "joins the patient's experience without the experience becoming part of the nurse's experience." A failure to maintain clear emotional boundaries between the patient and the nurse is likely to result in "vicarious trauma." Vicarious trauma may also be referred to as compassion fatigue, which often results from repeated exposure to hearing histories of trauma survivors.

Some researchers submit that vicarious trauma is an inevitable sequel to repeated exposure to trauma-focused interactions. Implications from these studies suggest the importance of self-care when repeatedly working with patients presenting with current or past histories of trauma.[23,24] Self-care activities include participating in support groups that focus on education about cumulative stress reactions in nurses and other providers, support from others sharing similar experiences, and stress management activities, such as regular exercise programs, healthy diets, sleep hygiene, and relaxation and deep breathing exercises.

### Trauma Awareness

Trauma awareness is a process in which the nurse's knowledge about trauma is used to conduct a comprehensive biopsychosocial assessment, assess acute and chronic symptoms and initiate trauma-specific interventions. Before conducting the initial assessment, it is imperative for underlying medical conditions that mimic psychiatric conditions (ie, mood and anxiety disorders) to be ruled out from history and physical examinations and diagnostic laboratory studies. Initial or acute traumatic stress symptoms include physiologic, emotional, cognitive, and behavioral reactions such as the following[1]:

- Intense anxiety, irritability or "edginess";
- Tearfulness or crying during examinations without obvious cause;
- Distancing or extreme quietness;
- Difficulty concentrating or answering questions, or being easily distracted;
- Marked emotional or startle reactions to seemingly nonthreatening interactions;
- Brief dissociation (ie, "losing it") and emotional numbness;
- Sleep disturbances; and
- Avoidance behaviors, isolation.

Given that trust is often a challenge for trauma survivors, it is imperative for the nurse to begin the assessment process by helping the patient to understand the screening process, reasons for asking specific questions, and the option of not answering questions. Observing the patient's reactions to questions can guide the pace and direction of the assessment process. Some patients may feel fearful or unsafe about sharing the traumatic experience and its aftermath. Awareness of emotional, cognitive, behavioral, and physiologic distress associated with trauma engenders a sense of security and safety throughout the evaluation process.

Although the initial reactions to the patient's traumatic experience may be intense and often stressful, additional aspects of the biopsychosocial assessment are equally important. A comprehensive biopsychosocial assessment includes a mental status examination; reasons for seeking treatment at this time; current and past psychiatric and medical treatments; quality of support systems and coping behaviors; assess sleeping disturbances, which are associated with prolonged trauma reactions; a present or past history of suicidal/homicidal ideations; current medications, including herbal and over-the-counter medications; and gender and cultural needs.

Traditional cultural beliefs and health practices vary among cultures, ethnicities, communities, families, and individuals. Thus, assessing the patient's cultural can be determined by assessment data concerning the role of healing practices, spiritual beliefs, health practices, societal and generational trauma and abuse, and quality of coping patterns, self-efficacy, social adjustment, resilience, optimism, and support.[25,26] Equally important is determining the patient's perception of how the family is responding and reacting to the current trauma and its impact on his or her self-esteem, self-efficacy skills, and recovery process. It is also necessary to rule out common coexisting psychiatric conditions associated with acute and chronic stress, such as depression, substance use disorders, and personality and anxiety disorders.

### Emphasize Safety

Maslow's hierarchy of needs[27] provides a basis for the discussion about personal safety for trauma survivors. According to his theory, once basic physiologic needs are met or satisfied, personal safety becomes a priority. In the case of traumatic events that threaten one's physical and mental integrity, personal safety is necessary to restore homeostasis and safety.[27] Safety begins with creating an accepting and nonjudgmental approach that helps the patient to recall the trauma knowing that safety measures are in place. Because of these intense emotional encounters, it important for the nurse initiate interventions that allay anxiety while asking the patient to recall the trauma and help him or her to refocus on the present. It is essential to use caution during these interactions because the patient may have difficulty distinguishing information that "triggered" the current reaction from the actual trauma and act as though the event is recurring. If the patient continues to have difficulty refocusing on the present, the nurse needs to stop the inquiry, offer support, and observe the patient's emotional, physical, and cognitive reactions. In addition, the nurse should seek consultation and collaboration with a mental health provider. In the event that the patient becomes more agitated and threatening, appropriate safety measures must be initiated. These grounding techniques are helpful in defusing overwhelming feelings and helping the patient return to the present or here and now[21,28–30] (**Box 2**).

### Strength-Based Care: Respect the Survivor's Input and Concerns in All Aspects of Care

Because this may be the survivor's first conversation about the trauma, it is critical for the nurse to provide privacy and safety and avoid interruptions, particularly when the patients expresses or exhibits intense emotional responses to questions about the traumatic event. It is also essential for the nurse to give full attention to and focus directly on the patient by using good eye contact and active listening skills and being mindful of one's own reactions to a difficult and possibly overwhelming emotional situation. Equally important is approaching the patient in a nonthreatening (ie, avoid sudden movements or touching, using a normal voice tone and maintaining ample personal space to avoid retraumatization; see **Box 1**).

---

**Box 2**
**Examples of grounding techniques**

- Open your eyes.
- Ask yourself. "What is my name? Who is in the room with me now?"
- Take slow deep breaths and pay attention to your breathing rate.
- Look around the room. What do you see, hear, smell, and feel?
- Focus on groupings, such as pets, colors, or cars.
- Think about a place where you felt was quiet, calm, and tranquil.
- Count from 1 to 10 slowly or repeat the alphabet.

*Data from* Refs.[28–30]

---

Throughout the initial assessment process and treatment planning, it is imperative to ask questions about the patient's preferences, wishes, abilities, and strengths. Strength-based approaches enable the nurse to acknowledge the patient holistically and implement individualized care. This process requires asking questions with the knowledge that some answers may be more difficult or painful than others. The nurse's personal experiences with resolved or unresolved trauma are likely to impede objectivity and impact how the nurse responds to the patient. Specifically, unresolved grief from personal trauma is likely to result in an inappropriate response from the nurse. Examples of these responses include either "overprotecting or rescuing the patient" or "intense reactions or distancing." Failure to recognize one's personal reactions in these situations can have an adverse effect on the nurse–patient relationship and impede the patient's recovery and healing. It is important for the nurse to reflect on personal reactions to the patient's experience and seek opportunities (ie, professional supervision, support group) to resolve personal feelings, thoughts, and beliefs about past trauma using healthy and adaptive coping skills that promote resilience and recovery.

### Offer Opportunities to Reclaim Control

Trauma survivors often feel vulnerable and exposed within themselves and in relationships with others. Helping the patient to reclaim control needs to be guided by the patient's readiness to regain personal control over painful memories and life. Findings from researchers examining the cognitive perspective of trauma exposure indicate that vulnerability to PTSD parallels the individual's ability to maintain a sense of control and self-efficacy and predictability during the trauma.[31]

Trauma survivors should be afforded opportunities to reclaim control regardless of where they seek treatment. It is important for psychiatric nurses to offer trauma survivors information about treatment options, collaborate in the development of their treatment plans, and facilitate self-efficacy. For instance, in the case of rape, the patient who seeks help in the emergency department may feel exposed when asked to remove clothing for a physical or other medical procedures. It is important for the nurse to assess for signs of anxiety and distress, explain all procedures, and ensure privacy, such as closing the curtains in the examination area. For many trauma survivors, these situations generate intense anxiety, fear of being touched or exposed, and a sense of powerlessness or loss of control. During these situations some patient's respirations and heart rate my increase owing to intense and anxiety and fears. Encouraging deep breathing exercises and stress management techniques can reduce these physiologic responses and help the patient to refocus on the examination and discuss concerns. In addition, giving choices, inquiring about the most comfortable position when a physical examination is required, and using same gender provider (ie, female provider with female patient) as requested.[32–34]

As the patient moves through the recovery process, treatment considerations must be based on collaboration with the patient and a host of providers. The following section provides a synopsis of treatment considerations for trauma and stress-related disorders.

## TREATMENT CONSIDERATIONS FOR TRAUMA AND STRESS-RELATED DISORDERS

Trauma and stress-related disorders that frequently coexist with psychiatric disorders, such as depression, anxiety, and substance use disorders, and medical disorders are challenging to treat. Research indicates that the complexity of these disorders requires a host of evidence-based treatment that integrates pharmacologic and psychotherapeutic approaches that facilitate recovery and address traumatic stress and coexisting disorders.[33] Trauma-focused cognitive behavioral therapies, such as prolonged exposure therapy or cognitive reprocessing therapy, have proven efficacy in the treatment of PTSD and other stress-related disorders.[35,36] For a synopsis of treatment considerations, see **Box 3** (see Deborah Antai-Otong: Anxiety Disorders: Treatment Considerations, in this issue for a comprehensive discussion of treatment considerations for PTSD).

---

**Box 3**
**Treatment considerations for trauma and stress-related disorders**

- *Psychopharmacologic*[37,38]: Manage coexisting psychiatric disorders (ie, depression, anxiety disorders) and obviate suicide risk.

- *Selective serotonin reuptake inhibitors*: Approved by the US Food and Drug Administration (ie, sertraline, paroxetine)

- *Prazosin*: Alpha adrenergic-blocking agents
  - Off-label for the treatment of nightmares and related sleep disturbance.

- Benzodiazepines should be avoided because they:
  - Only mitigate nonspecific anxiety and are unsuccessful in reducing core symptoms of posttraumatic stress disorder;
  - Increase the risk of addiction and dependence, as well as sedation and balance problems in older adults; and
  - May interfere with or disinhibit the psychological processes required to benefit from psychotherapies.

- Psychotherapeutic[35,36]:
  - Trauma-focused cognitive–behavioral therapy;
  - Exposure therapy;
  - Cognitive reprocessing;
  - Eye movement desensitization and reprocessing;
  - Stress inoculation training;
  - Mindfulness;
  - Yoga;
  - Psychoeducation; and
  - Sleep hygiene.

## SUMMARY

Although trauma exposure is common, few people will develop acute and chronic psychiatric disorders, such as PTSD. Those who develop PTSD are likely to have coexisting psychiatric and physical disorders and be high users of primary care and emergency departments. Psychiatric nurses are poised to lead their organizations in the implementation of trauma-informed care to ensure that trauma survivors safely transition through their journey of recovery to reclaim control over painful memories and their lives. Psychiatric nurses must be knowledgeable about trauma responses, implement evidence-based approaches to conduct comprehensive assessments, and create safe environments that help patients to modulate painful memories of their trauma.

A plethora of evidence-based pharmacologic and psychotherapeutic approaches are available to treat acute and chronic trauma and stress-related disorders. Although most researchers assert that trauma-focused cognitive–behavioral approaches demonstrate the most efficacious treatment outcomes, few studies demonstrate full symptom remission. New integrated approaches, such as using psychotherapy to facilitate cognitive training (ie, improving verbal memory) and pharmacologic treatments to manage nightmares and sleep disturbances (ie, prazosin) and coexisting depression and substance use disorder, offer promising treatment options to trauma survivors.

As a final point, repeated encounters with trauma survivors are extremely taxing and exhausting. During these stressful encounters, it is imperative for nurses to recognize personal reactions and initiate self-care techniques to mitigate the risk of vicarious trauma. This article provides an overview of salient clinical factors necessary to help the trauma survivor begin the process of healing and recovery and attain an optimal level of functioning.

## REFERENCES

1. American Psychiatric Association. Diagnostic and statistical manual of mental disorders. 5th edition. Washington, DC: Author; 2013.
2. Hager AD, Runtz MG. Physical and psychological maltreatment in childhood and later health problems in women: an exploratory investigation of the roles of perceived stress and coping strategies. Child Abuse Negl 2012;36:393–403.
3. Breslau N. Epidemiologic studies of trauma, posttraumatic stress disorder, and other psychiatric disorders. Can J Psychiatry 2002;47:923–9.
4. Kessler RC, Sonnega A, Bromet E, et al. Posttraumatic stress disorder in the National Comorbidity Survey. Arch Gen Psychiatry 1995;52:1048–60.
5. Bryant RA, Creamer M, O'Donnell M, et al. The capacity of acute stress disorder to predict posttraumatic psychiatric disorders. J Psychiatr Res 2012;46:168–73.
6. Manhapra A, Stefanovics E, Rosenheck R. Treatment outcomes for veterans with PTSD and substance use: impact of specific substances and achievement of abstinence. Drug Alcohol Depend 2015;156:70–7.
7. O'Donovan A, Cohen BE, Seal KH, et al. Elevated risk for autoimmune disorders in Iraq and Afghanistan veterans with posttraumatic stress disorder. Biol Psychiatry 2015;15:365–74.
8. Batty GD, Russ TC, Stamatakis E, et al. Psychological distress and risk of peripheral vascular disease, abdominal aortic aneurysm, and heart failure: pooling of sixteen cohort studies. Atherosclerosis 2014;236:385–8.
9. Pietzak RH, Goldstein RB, Southwick SM, et al. Medical comorbidity of full and partial posttraumatic stress disorder in US adults: results from Wave 2 of the

national epidemiologic survey on alcohol and related Conditions. Psychosom Med 2011;73:697–707.

10. Stein DJ, Chiu WT, Hwang I, et al. Cross-national analysis of the associations between traumatic events and suicidal behavior: findings from the WHO World Mental Health Surveys. PLoS One 2010;5:e1057.

11. Michopoulos V, Norrholm SD, Jovanovic T. Diagnostic biomarkers for posttraumatic stress disorder: promising horizons from translational neuroscience research. Biol Psychiatry 2015;78:344–53.

12. Guez J, Hertzanu-Lati M, Lev-Wiesel R, et al. Dissociative reality and dissociative being in therapy for post traumatic patients. Isr J Psychiatry Relat Sci 2015;52:47–53.

13. Perrin M, Vandeleur CL, Castelao E, et al. Determinants of the development of post-traumatic stress disorder, in the general population. Soc Psychiatry Psychiatr Epidemiol 2014;49:447–57.

14. Maier SF, Watkins LR. Role of the medial prefrontal cortex in coping and resilience. Brain Res 2010;1355:52–60.

15. Rajkumar R, Wu Y, Farooq U, et al. Stress activates the nucleus incertus and modulates plasticity in the hippocampo-medial prefrontal cortical pathway. Brain Res Bull 2015;120:83–9.

16. Farooq U, Rajkumar R, Sukumaran S, et al. Corticotropin-releasing factor infusion into nucleus incertus suppresses medial prefrontal cortical activity and hippocampo-medial prefrontal cortical long-term potentiation. Eur J Neurosci 2013;38:2516–25.

17. Kitamura T, Inokuchi K. Role of adult neurogenesis in hippocampal-cortical memory consolidation. Mol Brain 2014;7:13.

18. Powers A, Cross D, Fani N, et al. PTSD, emotion dysregulation, and dissociative symptoms in a highly traumatized sample. J Psychiatr Res 2015;61:174–9.

19. Bryant RA, Creamer M, O'Donnell M, et al. A comparison of the capacity of DSM-IV and DSM-5 acute stress disorder definitions to predict posttraumatic stress disorder and related disorders. J Clin Psychiatry 2015;76:391–7.

20. Hopper EK, Bassuk EL, Olivet J. Shelter from the storm: trauma-informed care in homelessness services settings. Open Health Serv Policy J 2010;2010(3):80–100.

21. Substance Abuse and Mental Health Services Administration. Trauma-informed care in behavioral health services. Treatment improvement protocol (TIP) series 57. HHS publication No. (SMA). Rockville (MD): Substance Abuse and Mental Health Services Administration; 2014.

22. Raja S, Hasnain M, Hoersch M, et al. Trauma informed care in medicine: current knowledge and future research directions. Fam Community Health 2015;38:216–26.

23. Tabor PD. Vicarious traumatization: concept analysis. J Forensic Nurs 2011;7:203–8.

24. Bellolio MF, Cabrera D, Sadosty AT, et al. Compassion fatigue is similar in emergency medicine residents compared to other medical and surgical specialties. West J Emerg Med 2014;15:629–35.

25. Gone JP. Reconsidering American Indian historical trauma: lessons from an early Gros Ventre war narrative. Transcult Psychiatry 2014;51:387–406.

26. Cloud RL, Hammack PL. Surviving colonization and the quest for healing: narrative and resilience among California Indian tribal leaders. Transcult Psychiatry 2014;51:112–33.

27. Maslow AH. A theory of human motivation. Psychol Rev 1943;50:370–96.

28. Reeves E. A synthesis of the literature on trauma-informed care. Issues Ment Health Nurs 2015;36:698–709.
29. Najavits L. Seeking Safety: a treatment manual for PTSD and substance abuse. Using grounding to detach from emotional pain. New York: Guildford Press; 2002. p. 133–5.
30. Brier J, Scott C. Principles of trauma therapy: a guide to symptoms, evaluation, and treatment. 2nd edition. Thousand Oaks (CA): Sage Publications; 2012.
31. Brown AD, Joscelyne A, Dorfman ML, et al. The impact of perceived self-efficacy on memory for aversive experiences. Memory 2012;20:374–83.
32. Mason R, O'Rinn SE. Co-occurring intimate partner violence, mental health, and substance use problems: a scoping review. Glob Health Action 2014;7:24815, eCollection 2014.
33. Myers US, Browne KC, Norman SB. Treatment engagement: female survivors of intimate partner violence in treatment for PTSD and alcohol use disorder. J Dual Diagn 2015;11:238–47.
34. Peri T, Gofman M, Tal S, et al. Embodied simulation in exposure-based therapies for posttraumatic stress disorder-a possible integration of cognitive behavioral theories, neuroscience, and psychoanalysis. Eur J Psychotraumatol 2015;6:29301.
35. Cusack K, Jonas DE, Forneris CA, et al. Psychological treatments for adults with posttraumatic stress disorder: a systematic review and meta-analysis. Clin Psychol Rev 2016;43:128–41.
36. Steenkamp MM, Litz BT, Hoge CW, et al. Psychotherapy for military-related PTSD: a review of randomized clinical trials. JAMA 2015;314:489–500.
37. Beradis D, Manni S, Serroni N, et al. Targeting the noradrenergic system In posttraumatic stress disorder: a systematic review and meta-analysis of prazosin trials. Curr Drug Targets 2015;16:1094–106.
38. Hoskins M, Pearce J, Bethell A, et al. Pharmacotherapy for post-traumatic stress disorder: systematic review and meta-analysis. Br J Psychiatry 2015;206:93–100.

# Contemporary Treatment Approaches to Major Depression and Bipolar Disorders

Richard L. John Jr, MSN, PMHNP-BC, FNP-BC[a],*,
Deborah Antai-Otong, MS, APRN, PMHCNS-BC, FAAN[b]

## KEYWORDS

- Unipolar depression • Bipolar disorder • Antidepressants • Mood stabilizers
- Stressors • Suicide • Cognitive behavioral therapy

## KEY POINTS

- Mood disorders are common, recurring psychiatric disorders that are associated with nonadherence to treatment and when left untreated are contributors to physical morbidity and mortality.
- Mood disorders have a high incidence of coexisting psychiatric, substance use, and physical disorders.
- Unipolar and bipolar disorders are linked to vast chronic physical disorders (ie, cancer, diabetes, immunologic disorders).
- A comprehensive biopsychosocial assessment, precluded by medical assessment, is critical to determine a definitive diagnosis.
- Evidence-based treatment for mood disorders includes pharmacotherapy and psychotherapeutic interventions that are governed by person-centered, strength, and recovery-based principles.

## INTRODUCTION

Mood disorders are common and recurrent psychiatric disorders. Unipolar or major depressive and bipolar disorders are major categories of mood disorders. Major depressive episodes in each category refer to a sad or depressed mood and alterations in concentration, appetite, sleeping patterns, and functional performance.[1] In comparison, manic episodes manifest as expanded, elated, or irritable mood; decreased need for

Disclosure Statement: The authors have nothing to disclose.
This article is an update of an article previously published in Nursing Clinics of North America, Volume 38, Issue 1, March 2003.
[a] Department of Veterans Affairs-Greater Los Angeles, 11301 Wilshire Boulevard, Los Angeles, CA 90073, USA; [b] Department of Veterans Affairs, Veterans Integrated Service Networks-(VISN-17), 2301 E. Lamar Boulevard, Arlington, TX 76006, USA
* Corresponding author.
E-mail address: Richard.JohnJr@va.gov

sleep; racing thoughts; inflated self-esteem; and pressured speech.[1] Overall mood disorders have become important contributors to morbidity and mortality related to coexisting physical disorders and suicide risk.[2,3] The high morbidity and mortality of mood disorders are frequently linked to nonadherence to medications. Nonadherence to a treatment regimen is significantly high in patients with mood disorders, particularly those with bipolar disorders. When left untreated or unrecognized, mood disorders are likely to impact quality of life and functionality and contribute to deleterious clinical outcomes. Given the enormity of deleterious clinical outcomes associated with mood disorders, early identification of individuals at risk for coexisting psychiatric, substance use, and physical disorders must be a health care priority.

### Prevalence

According to the World Health Organization,[2] major depression is one of most common psychiatric disorders and carries the highest burden of disability among all psychiatric disorders. The prevalence of mood disorders transcends race, ethnicity, socioeconomic class, gender, and age. The onset of depression is around 25 years of age in Western countries, and women are more likely to experience depression than men.[4] Gender, life span, hormonal and environmental factors, and psychosocial- and trauma-related events purportedly expand the risk of depression in women. Significant personal losses, coexisting physical disorders, cognitive deficits, social isolation, life satisfaction, and adjustment to aging are associated with depression in older adults.[5]

Twin and family studies indicate that mood disorders are highly heritable and run in some families. Brain imaging studies implicate alterations in neuroanatomical brain structures and functions in the genesis of unipolar and bipolar disorders.[6] Environmental and psychosocial factors and gender are also linked to the origins of mood disorders. These underpinnings are principal biomarkers and treatment targets and are believed to underlie the onset, maintenance, and recurrence of mood disorders.[7]

Consistent data from large epidemiologic studies point a 1% prevalence of bipolar I disorder and an additional 3% for bipolar II disorder.[4,8,9] Data from the National Comorbidity Study indicate a lifetime prevalence of about 4% for bipolar disorder. Symptoms of bipolar disorder usually emerge in adolescence or early adulthood and rarely in late adulthood.[10] Bipolar disorder is more prevalent in women than men at a ratio of 3:2. The average age for women to have bipolar disorder diagnosed is 25 years and earlier in men. According to researchers, major gender differences in the bipolar disorders include an earlier onset and coexisting substance use disorders (ie, alcohol use) in men compared with higher rates of depression and coexisting psychiatric disorders in women.[11] Concurrent psychiatric, substance use, and physical disorders are more the rule than the exception in patients with bipolar disorder.[12] Similar to unipolar depression, bipolar disorders consume enormous health care resources, but they are more costly in patients with bipolar disorders.[13] A large percentage of patients with mood disorders seek health care services through primary care settings.[14] The high prevalence of patients seeking these services in primary care makes it critical for providers to accurately discern symptoms of mood disorders and coexisting disorders to ensure early and appropriate treatment. High health care costs, including failure to collaborate with a mental health professional and monitor treatment responses, are owing to the impact of these disorders on functional, physical, psychosocial, cognitive and occupational impairment. According to researchers, patients with mood disorders seek services in several health care settings, and average time to receive initial treatment is 10 years. The high incidence of these disorders also contributes to the alarming suicide risk in this population.[2,3,15] Timely recognition, accurate diagnosis, and appropriate treatment can reduce health care utilization and adverse consequences associated with mood disorders.

Despite the availability of vast treatment options, mood disorders are difficult to treat and sustain symptom remission. This is particularly evident in patients with bipolar disorders because of the dynamic and unstable course of this disorder and high prevalence of nonadherence to medication regimen. Researchers submit that nonadherence to medication is the greatest predictor of adverse and poor clinical outcomes.[13,16]

This article provides an overview of evidence-based care of patients with unipolar and bipolar disorders. Causative factors of mood disorders, the importance of medical clearance, and the use of a comprehensive biopsychosocial assessment are also reviewed. This article discusses the importance of the psychiatric nurse in establishing collaborative relationships with patients and their families to develop person-centered treatment that facilitates optimal functioning and quality of life.

## CAUSES OF MOOD DISORDERS

The precise cause of unipolar or major depressive disorders remains an enigma despite decades of studies searching for unique biomarkers as treatment targets. A comprehensive review of major underpinnings of mood disorders is beyond the scope of this article. However, a quick overview of salient points about causative factors is presented in the following section.

### Unipolar Depression

Converging data from numerous studies indicate the role of genetics, gender, alterations in diverse neurotransmitters, the hypothalamic pituitary-adrenal axis that mediates stress hormones, and structural and functional defects as major causes of depression. Twin studies related to genetic vulnerability and familial patterns are widely accepted as prominent contributors to the genesis of mood disorders. Genetic factors are believed to be mediated by environmental factors and heighten the vulnerability of depression.[17]

Purportedly, norepinephrine, serotonin, and dopamine, neurotransmitters located primarily in the amygdala, hippocampal, limbic, and frontal cortical areas mediate intricate neural pathways that regulate feelings, thoughts, mood, and behavior and modulate stress and cognitive functioning.[18] Depletion of these neurochemicals is implicated in the genesis of unipolar depressive disorders. Supposedly, antidepressants increase the levels of these neurochemicals and produce improved mood and function. However, the precise mechanism for these actions is not clearly understood and continues to be researched.

Newer data implicate that the pathogenesis and treatment of depression is associated with alterations in additional neural circuits, such glutamatergic mechanisms.[19] The glutamatergic neurotransmitter system continues to be studied as a possible basis for discovering newer antidepressants. Emerging evidence implicates the antidepressant effects of newer agents to their ability to produce neuroplasticity changes that improve symptoms of depression. Ketamine, a glutamate receptor antagonist is an example of these drugs. Researchers assert that low-dose ketamine has a more rapid onset when compared with older antidepressants that require 8 to 12 weeks to demonstrate their efficacy.[19] Newer agents continue to be researched and in the future will offer additional options for major depressive disorder.

Consistent findings from neuroimaging studies show that patients with unipolar depression have abnormalities in several areas including the limbic-anterior cingulate prefrontal neural circuitry, dorsolateral prefrontal cortex, and medical prefrontal cortex.[6,20] These brain regions and neurocircuitries play key roles in emotional processing and modulation of stress.

The precise cause of unipolar depression is multifaceted. However, the aforementioned factors are mediated by environmental, genetics, gender, and neurochemical factors and underlie clinical symptoms of these mood disorders.

## Bipolar Disorders

Although unipolar and bipolar disorders are both mood disorders there are differences in the genesis of symptoms and treatment considerations. Confounding evidence implicates various neuroanatomic brain structures in the genesis of bipolar disorder. The most consistent findings from neuroimaging studies implicate increased activation and alterations in the left amygdala and frontal-limbic regions and reduced activation of the right dorsolateral prefrontal cortex. These regions are believed to cause major symptoms of mania.[21] More specifically, abnormalities in these brain regions underlie cognitive, emotional, and sleep lability in patients with bipolar disorder that persist regardless of manic, hypomanic, or depressed or euthymic state.[22–24] These biomarkers are also target sites for pharmacotherapies used to treat individuals with bipolar disorder.

The distinction between depressive episodes in unipolar and bipolar disorders continues to challenge psychiatric nurses and other providers in making differential diagnoses that ensure the patient receives appropriate treatment. Because of the high incidence of co-occurring psychiatric, substance use, and physical disorders in the patient with a mood disorder, the nurse must rule out these conditions and begin this process with medical clearance.

## Medical Assessment

Medical assessment is a critical component to making an accurate diagnosis of mood disorders and initiating appropriate treatment considerations. Caring for patients with mood disorders begins with making an accurate diagnosis based on the findings from a comprehensive history and physical examination. This process requires a host of diagnostic studies including vitamin B12 and folate levels and hematologic, renal and hepatic, endocrine, and cardiovascular studies, including electrocardiogram, pregnancy test, and drug screens. Several medical conditions mimic symptoms of mood disturbances, such as thyroid disorders (ie, hyper- or hypothyroidism), medication side effects, fluid and electrolyte disturbances (ie, delirium), diabetes, drug toxicity, and early stages of neurocognitive disorders, particularly when there is a gradual decline in cognitive function (ie, Alzheimer disease).[5] Of particular importance is the differential diagnosis of dementia and depression, particularly in older adults with cognitive deficits. Cognitive deficits in older adults may be the initial symptoms of neurocognitive disorders.[5] When medical clearance is confirmed, the nurse can integrate this information into the biopsychosocial assessment.

## Biopsychosocial Assessment

Similar to various means of data collection and analyses the biopsychosocial assessment process begins with establishing a therapeutic relationship that builds trust and conveys empathy. Creating a safe environment enables the nurse to gather important information about the history of the onset, frequency and severity of symptoms, and current and past treatment and assess the patient's coping skills associated with managing stressful situations. When questioning about the severity of symptoms, it is important to discuss their impact on personal, functional, and occupational performance and interpersonal relationships, Also, an accepting and nonjudgmental approach helps the nurse glean a greater understanding of the patient's experience of his or her symptoms, insight into treatment choices, and the importance of medication adherence. It is critical for the nurse to corroborate the patient's history of symptoms, adherence to treatment regimens, and related behaviors with family members and significant others. Conducting a mental status examination and ongoing suicide risk assessment are critical components of the evaluation process.

Major aspects of a biopsychosocial assessment include:

- Reasons for seeking treatment at this time
- Chief complaint
- Duration and course of symptoms (ie, history of highs or manic episodes— important data to help rule out unipolar vs bipolar depression and treatment considerations)
- Current and past treatment for psychiatric (ie, hospitalizations) substance use disorders, including smoking and gambling, and physical disorders
- History of adherence to treatment, including medications; reasons for nonadherence (ie, side effects); and psychotherapy (ie, expensive, ineffective)
- History of adverse effects from medications and other treatment regimens
- Trauma history that includes the physical, emotional, and sexual traumas from childhood as well as date rape, deaths of friends and family, and other accidents— all traumas that can all contribute to the combined exposure and risk of depression
- History of violence toward self and others
- Nature of presence of suicidal thoughts, plan, and intent, recent/past attempts, and related stressors
  - Family history of suicide and self-destructive behaviors, including attempts, and relationship to family members(s) (See Jeffery Ramirez: Suicide: Across the Life Span, in this issue on Suicide for additional discussion about the assessment of the patient at risk for suicide.)
  - Family history of mania and irritable mood states
- History of hormonal mood changes across the life span before or during menses, pregnancy, postpartum, perimenopause, and menopause
- Military history and experience, including combat and military sexual trauma
- Substance use history, including type, duration of use, treatment, legal impact (ie, arrests, probation/parole, convictions), occupational performance (ie, employment history), interpersonal relationships, and last use
- Current medications, including prescribed, over the counter, and herbal and dietary supplements with psychoactive properties
- Dietary habits and regular wellness activities
- Medical history, allergies
- Family, personal, social, occupational history
- Social habits, such as drugs, alcohol, gambling, smoking
- Spiritual, cultural, religious and related health practices.

## Mental Status Examination

A basic mental status examination includes a general description of the patient's:

- Demeanor
- Appropriateness of dress, hygiene, and personal appearance
- Eye contact (consider cultural factors)
- Level of consciousness
- Level and quality of engagement with nurse and family members
- Quality and rate of speech and thought processes

- Mood congruence
- Psychomotor performance and functioning

### Suicide Risk Assessment

There is an inherent risk of suicide in all patients with psychiatric disorders but especially in those with a mood disorder. The incidence is even greater in this population because of the high incidence of coexisting psychiatric, substance use, and physical disorders.[2,3] Although the precise predication of suicide is unknown, psychiatric mental health nurses must conduct initial and ongoing suicide risk assessments on all patients regardless of the diagnosis. The Substance Abuse and Mental Health Services[25] has developed a 5-step suicide risk assessment tool that can assist in the identification of patients at risk for suicide. Three components of this tool are high-risk factors (**Box 1**), protective factors (**Box 2**), and documentation.[25]

### Documentation

When a patient is identified as high risk, it is imperative for the nurse to initiate interventions that mitigate risk and ensure patient safety. Normally, interventions include one-to-one observations and brief hospitalization. When documenting the care of a patient who is considered at risk for suicide it is important to document all clinical

---

**Box 1**
**High-risk factors**

- American Indian/Alaskan Native
- Depression or bereavement
- Previous attempts
- Discharged from inpatient psychiatric services within last 4 weeks
- Hopelessness, isolation, feeling trapped
- Intoxication—alcohol and other drugs
- Gender and age
- Recently widowed
- Access to firearms, bridges, buildings and railroads, poisonous gases, and medications
- Personality disorder, (eg, impulsivity)
- Living alone, divorced, social withdrawn
- Unemployment
- Acute psychosis
- Health status—physical and or debilitating illness, chronic pain
- Loss, relationship breakup
- Family chaos, sense of isolation
- Worsening physical conditions, including chronic pain
- History of physical or sexual abuse and other trauma
- Genetic and biological factors (eg, low serotonin, psychiatric conditions, family history)
- Societal stigma attached to help-seeking behaviors

*Data from* Refs.[25,30,41]

| Box 2 |
| --- |
| **Protective factors across all populations** |

- Reasons for living
- Children in the home
- Religious and spiritual beliefs
- Employment
- Optimism and hope
- Connectedness to individuals, family, community, and social institutions
- Ethnic and cultural factors
- Cultural identification
- Reality testing ability
- Positive coping and problem-solving skills
- Positive and strong social support
- Access to mental health care

*Data from* U.S. Department of Health and Human Services: substance abuse and mental health services administration HHS Publication No. (SMA) 09-4432 • CMHS-NSP-0193. 2009. Available at: http://store.samhsa.gov/product/Suicide-Assessment-Five-Step-Evaluation-and-Triage-SAFE-T-Pocket-Card-for-Clinicians/SMA09-4432; and Centers for Disease Control and Prevention. Suicide among adults aged 35–64 years–United States, 1999–2010. MMWR Morb Mortal Wkly Rep 2013;62:1–24. Available at: http://www.cdc.gov/mmwr/preview/mmwrhtml/mm6217a1.htm. Accessed December 27, 2015.

actions to create a medical and legal account of the client's care and include the following:

- What information did the nurse obtain, ie, risk assessment and rationale for clinical decisions?
- When and what actions were taken to mitigate risk factors?
- How did the nurse follow up on the patient's treatment and suicidal thoughts and behaviors?
- Who was given the hand-off and referral?[26]

(For an in-depth approach related to caring for patients at risk for suicide, including the development, use and documentation of a safety plan, see Jeffery Ramirez: Suicide: Across the Life Span, in this issue).

Overall, data analysis from the comprehensive biopsychosocial assessment is critical in making an accurate diagnosis of mood disorders. A definitive diagnosis is based on criteria established by the American Psychiatric Association Diagnostic Manual of Mental Disorders, 5th edition (DSM-5).[1]

## DIAGNOSIS
### Major Depressive Disorder (Unipolar Depression)

The DSM-5,[1] describes major depressive disorder as a constellation of symptoms that lasts for at least 2 weeks, is not the patient's normal behavior, and includes at least depressed mood and loss of interest or pleasure and at least 5 of the following occurring daily or nearly every day:

- Sad or depressed mood
- Lack of interest in activities that were previously pleasurable

- Significant change in weight or appetite
- Substantial observable change in activity level, increased or decreased or early morning awakenings, or lack of restful sleep
- Significant change in sleep pattern either increased or decreased
- Decreased energy level or fatigue
- Restlessness or pacing
- Slowed thinking, concentration or memory disturbances (ie, forgetfulness), difficulty remembering details and making decisions
- Thoughts of death or suicide or plans or attempts of self-harm

Collectively, these symptoms must cause significant difficulties to their ability to function at work, home, or social situations.[1]

### Persistent Depressive Disorder

Persistent depressive disorder[1] is a new DSM-5 category that combines dysthymic and chronic depression. Criteria for this disorder are unipolar disorder except for the duration. Typically, the symptoms of persistent depressive disorder persist for at least 2 years, and the patient is never symptom free for less than 2 months.

### Postpartum Depression

Postpartum depression (PPD) is more than the normal postpartum blues and normally the onset of symptoms is within 4 weeks after birth.[1] Some women have more severe symptoms of delusions that may present as overworrying about the safety of the newborn or fears of killing the infant. Timely treatment is critical to reducing harm to the infant and mother. Studies suggest that the risk of recurrent PPD postdelivery ranges from 30% to 50%. For these reasons, it is important to initiate preventive interventions to reduce the initial incidence of this disorder. Adverse consequences of postpartum depression include interference with the maternal role of bonding and responsive caregiving and protecting the child from harm (ie, vaccinations).[27,28] It is widely recognized that maternal-child bonding is important for the infant's neurodevelopment, mental health, and healthy relationships. Psychiatric nurses must collaborate with obstetrics/gynecology providers and pediatricians to assess the needs of women with depression before and after delivery and implement an integrated model of care for adolescents and adult women with PPD. The breadth of this topic extends beyond the capacity of this report, but, similar to other psychiatric disorders, conducting timely assessments is important; determining an accurate diagnosis and initiating appropriate treatment are critical in caring for women that present with PPD and their newborns.

### Seasonal Affective Disorder

Seasonal affective disorder is a recurring major depressive disorder whose symptoms of sad mood, fatigue, and increased appetite coincide with a seasonal pattern, such as fall and winter months when there is less exposure to sunlight. Symptoms recur over a 2-year period and remit typically during spring and summer months.[1] Similar to unipolar depression, the prevalence of seasonal affective disorder is higher in women than men. Treatment considerations include antidepressants, light therapy, and cognitive behavioral therapy.[29]

Overall, the treatment of mood disorders is manifold and determined by the definitive diagnosis of unipolar or a bipolar disorder. Positive clinical outcomes correlate with person-centered, strength, and recovery-based approaches that take into considerations the patient's wishes and preferences. Additional factors include age; gender; pregnancy and postpartum issues (ie, breast feeding); coexisting psychiatric, substance use, and medical disorders; family history; previous treatment response; and severity of symptoms.[30]

## TREATMENT CONSIDERATIONS FOR UNIPOLAR DEPRESSION (MAJOR DEPRESSIVE DISORDER)

Treatment considerations for unipolar or major depressive disorders during the acute phase include pharmacotherapy, psychotherapeutic approaches, and other somatic approaches. Because of the high incidence of suicide during this period, it is essential to monitor the patient for suicide risk throughout treatment.

Pharmacotherapy is widely accepted as the first-line treatment for major depressive episodes. Antidepressants are generally prescribed for patients presenting with a definitive diagnosis of major depressive episode. The most commonly prescribed categories of antidepressants are selective serotonin reuptake inhibitors and serotonin norepinephrine reuptake inhibitors (SNRI). Other antidepressants include venlafaxine, bupropion, mirtazapine, trazodone, tricyclic antidepressants (TCAs), and monoamine oxidase inhibitors (MAOIs) (**Table 1**). An exhaustive description of medications used in the treatment of major depressive disorder is beyond the scope of this article. (See Courtney J. Givens: Adverse Drug Reactions Associated with Antipsychotic, Antidepressants, Mood Stabilizers, and Stimulants, in this issue.)

According to the American Psychiatric Association's Practice Guidelines for the Treatment of Patients with Major Depressive Disorder,[30] the nurse prescriber should consider the following before initiating pharmacotherapy:

- Patient choice
- Previous response to treatment
- Medication efficacy and effectiveness
- Tolerability and likely side effects
- Risk of drug-to-drug interactions, particularly with coexisting psychiatric, substance use, and physical disorders
- Drug half-life[30]

The American Psychological Association (2010) delineates 3 phases of treatment for individuals with major depressive disorders: acute, continuation, and maintenance. During the acute phase, primary treatment goals include symptom remission and return to an optimal level of functioning and quality of life. Remission is defined as an absence of symptoms and it is correlated with a higher level of functioning, improved quality of life, and a better prognosis compared with poor or no remission.[30] Typically, symptom remission means that there is at least a 50% reduction in baseline symptoms as measured by standardized tools, such as the Hamilton Depression Rating Scale.[31] Remission is further described as sustained symptom remission over a 3-week period of sustained improved mood and interest in things once considered pleasurable and the absence of 3 or fewer of the remaining symptoms.[30] Symptom remission is likely to occur within 6 to 8 weeks of initiation of treatment. However, this period varies and is governed by manifold factors, including medication adherence, individual response to a given medication regimen, and severity of symptoms.[30]

During all phases of treatment, but particularly during the acute phase, the patient needs to be monitored regularly for symptom remission, suicide risk, side effects, signs of mania, and evidence of adherence to treatment.[30] Emergence of mania often indicates that the patient has either bipolar I or II depressive episode rather than unipolar depression and requires medications for bipolar disorders.

**Table 1**
**Common antidepressants and average doses**

| Antidepressant | Type | Average Dose[a] |
|---|---|---|
| Citalopram | SSRI | 40 mg |
| Escitalopram | SSRI | 20 mg |
| Fluoxetine | SSRI | 20 mg |
| Fluvoxamine | SSRI | 100 mg |
| Paroxetine | SSRI | 30 mg |
| Sertraline | SSRI | 100 mg |
| Clomipramine | TCA | 100 mg |
| Nortriptyline | TCA | 50 mg |
| Amitriptyline | TCA | 100 mg |
| Imipramine | TCA | 75 mg |
| Maprotiline | TCA | 75 mg |
| Desipramine | TCA | 75 mg |
| Trimipramine | TCA | 75 mg |
| Phenelzine | MAOi | 30 mg |
| Tranylcypromine | MAOi | 10 mg |
| Selegiline patch | MAOi | 6 mg |
| Selegiline | MAOi | 20 mg |
| Venlafaxine | SNRI | 150 mg |
| Duloxetine | SNRI | 60 mg |
| Desvenlafaxine | SNRI | 100 mg |
| Trazodone | Other | 200 mg |
| Nefazodone | Other | 400 mg |
| Bupropion | Other | 300 mg |
| Mirtazapine | Other | 30 mg |

[a] As typically prescribed.

The continuation phase occurs once the patient achieves symptom remission.[30] The principal goal of this phase, which about lasts 4 to 9 months, is the prevention of recurrence. Ideally, during this phase, the patient achieves a therapeutic level of medication with an absence of depressive symptoms and returns to and maintains a baseline level of functioning and quality of life.

During the maintenance phase, treatment involves continued medication and appointments to monitor response and identify early symptoms of recurrent depression.[30] Consistent data indicate that about only one-third of patients taking antidepressants actually achieve full remission. Data from the 2006 publication STAR*D (Sequenced Treatment Alternative to Relieve Depression) reported that only a third of the patients taking antidepressants had full remission from depressive symptoms and that 50% of these patients experienced half reduction in depressive symptoms after up to 14 weeks of antidepressant treatment.[3,31,32] When the patient has partial remission or poor response to antidepressant medications, the prescribing provider often initiates adjunct treatment (ie, second-generation antipsychotic) or switches to another antidepressant and psychotherapeutic interventions, such as cognitive behavioral therapy, psychoeducation, and family therapy. Severe forms of major depressive disorders (ie, psychotic symptoms or nonresponse to medication) may require somatic treatments, such as electroconvulsive therapy (ECT).

Patients who are poor responders to antidepressants must be assessed for nonadherence to medication regimen, to see if an adequate dose of medication is prescribed, and to see if the side effects are intolerable. Patients must be assessed for medication adherence either by serum levels when indicated or pill counts. Inquiring about side effects is equally important and should be explored during meetings with the patient and corroborated by family members. It should be determined if the medication dose is adequate or if it needs to be increased or changed, if the patient should be switched to another antidepressant, or if a second-generation antipsychotic should be added. Finally, other integrated treatments (ie, cognitive behavioral therapy) should be explored.[3,31,32]

Although pharmacotherapy is the mainstay treatment of mood disorders, a large percentage of patients never fully achieves remission. As such, treatment considerations need to include nonpharmacologic approaches such as psychotherapies, psychoeducation, and family intervention; somatic and complementary therapies; and alternative therapies.

### Psychotherapeutic Interventions

Cognitive behavioral therapies (CBT)[33] are the most widely studied psychotherapeutic approaches in the treatment of psychiatric disorders, such as depression, anxiety, and posttraumatic stress disorders. Depression is believed to be associated with negative or distorted thoughts, feelings, and behaviors, which are targets for cognitive behavioral therapy and pharmacologic interventions. Medications are used to reduce physiologic symptoms related to depression, such as fatigue, and cognitive deficits that interfere with learning new information and using principles of CBT. Key tenets of CBT involve one's primary beliefs about self, others, and the future.[33] These beliefs govern one's thoughts, feelings behaviors, and mood. Depression often indicates that the patient feels helpless and has negative and often distorted thoughts about self, others, and the world, such as "I lost my job," I am a failure, I will never be able to find another job." CBT allows the nurse psychotherapist to educate the patient about CBT, including how negative thoughts generate depression and anxiety. The patient uses these techniques to develop adaptive coping skills to realistically address life situations and challenge overgeneralizations and negative assumptions about self, others, and the world.

Homework assignments involve using real-life experiences to test these assumptions and dampen the patient's anxiety-provoking thoughts, feelings, and behaviors. Collectively, these activities promote adaptive coping skills and reduce feelings of helplessness.[33,34] (For a comprehensive discussion of major theories and concepts of CBT and their applicability to depressive and anxiety disorders see Deborah Antai-Otong: Anxiety Disorders: Treatment Considerations, in this issue.)

### Other Somatic Therapies

Despite proven efficacy of CBT and psychopharmacologic interventions, somatic treatment remains an option for the patient with a major depressive disorder. Of these approaches, ECT is considered the mainstay treatment of major depressive disorder when rapid response and remission are required, such as in patients who are severely depressed with psychotic features and at high risk for suicide.[35] Common side effects linked to ECT include memory difficulties (ie, retrograde) and a high prevalence of relapse without continuation. Additional clinical implications for ECT include catatonia, pregnancy, poor response to antidepressant medications, and serious medical disorders that prohibit the use of antidepressant medications.[30,35] In a recent study of the use of ECT during pregnancy, Leiknes and colleagues[36] asserted that this treatment modality should be used cautiously and as the last alternative for the treatment of depression; it should be grounded in sound clinical judgment because of potential negative outcomes.[37]

Deep brain stimulation, vagal nerve stimulation, and transcranial magnetic stimulation are newer somatic interventions. Typically, these interventions have shown modest improvement as monotherapy in the management of treatment-resistant depression. However, few clinical trials have been conducted to determine the long-term benefits of these approaches.[38,39]

### Complementary and Alternative Therapies

There is a growing public interest and popularity in the use of complementary and alternative therapies for treatment of depression. The most popular therapies include high-dose folic acid, vitamin D, omega-3-fatty acids, acupuncture, yoga, melatonin, and light therapy. There is a dearth of evidence supporting the efficacy of these remedies. St. John's Wort (hypericum perforatum) and SAMe (S-adenosyl-L-methionine) are examples of over-the-counter herbal preparations used to manage mild-to-moderate depression. It is important for patients to consult with their provider before taking these preparations and prescribed antidepressants.

Lastly, determining the best treatment modality for mood disorders requires collaboration between the psychiatric mental health nurse provider, the patient, and other providers. As more and more patients suffer from depression and seek treatment in primary care settings, it is critical for psychiatric mental health nurses to familiarize themselves with these complex disorders. The following discussion focuses on clinical symptoms and treatment considerations for bipolar I and bipolar II disorders.

### Bipolar Disorders

Bipolar disorders differ from unipolar depressive disorder because the former includes a history of cyclic mania, hypomania, or mixed states. According to researchers, clinical features of bipolar disorders are determined by the incidence of or cycling between manic and depressive episodes.[1,9] Similar to unipolar disorder, bipolar disorders are associated with a high incidence of coexisting psychiatric, substance use, and physical disorders (ie, cardiovascular and metabolic conditions), such as attention deficit hyperactivity disorder and personality disorders (ie, borderline personality disorder).[1]

### Bipolar I Disorder

According to the DSM-5[1] there are 2 distinct poles or phases of bipolar disorders that include both depressed and manic phases. The criteria for bipolar disorder include the depressed episode symptoms and symptoms of a lifetime history of at least one manic episode. Symptoms of bipolar disorders may appear identical to major depression in its depressed phase. For many patients, the lack of recollection of their manic episode into their disorders and minimization of symptom severity can impede the early diagnosis of bipolar disorders. If the manic phase is not identified, unipolar depression is most likely diagnosed. The symptoms that identify a manic episode include the following:

- Physical arousal with excessive energy and activity, restlessness
- Emotional lability, mood swings (ie, mania, agitation, irritability)
- Rapid and pressured speech, racing thoughts, overthinking situations or ideas
- Sleep disturbances and the decreased need for sleep
- Grandiose delusions or thoughts of self-importance

- Disregard for the physical or financial consequences in personal, social, and business encounters.
- These symptoms must last for at least 1 week, unless hospitalized, and cause a significant disruption in the persons social or occupational functioning.[1]

### Bipolar II Disorder

Bipolar II disorder involves recurrent episodes of hypomania and major depression but not a full manic episode, as listed above. The duration aspect is only 4 days and not a full week of symptoms. An important change to DSM-5 is the inclusion of activity and energy level and mood level in the diagnosis. Under the DSM-5, the mood criterion now includes hopelessness. There can be no previous symptoms of psychosis for this diagnosis, which becomes an exclusionary factor. Because of similarities between unipolar major depressive disorder and bipolar types I and II, providers may misdiagnosis the condition as the former and initiate antidepressants. Psychiatric nurse prescribers must monitor for signs of a manic episode when the patient is determined to have a diagnosis of unipolar depression. Likewise, when asking patients about hypomania, a distinction between increased energy associated with an antidepressant and a full history of these symptoms must be carefully assessed.[1]

The hypomania episode must last for most of the day, every day, for at least 4 days. In addition, 3 or more of the following symptoms will be present.

- Decreased need for sleep
- More talkative
- Subjective experience of thoughts/ideas racing
- Distractibility
- Increase in goal-directed activity or psychomotor agitation
- Excessive involvement in pleasurable activities with a high potential of painful consequences
- Negative history of a manic, hypomanic, or mixed episode[1]

### Pharmacologic Interventions

The most commonly used medications for bipolar disorders include mood stabilizers, such as lithium; anticonvulsant agents, such as lamotrigine; and most of the second-generation antipsychotics, such as quietiapine.[13,15,39] Acute mania is normally treated in the emergency room or an acute inpatient psychiatric setting with a parenteral conventional antipsychotic agent, such as haloperidol and benzodiazepine, or second-generation antipsychotic agent. Mood stabilizers such as lithium or anticonvulsants are titrated over at least a 2-week period or until a therapeutic serum level is reached or symptom remission is attained (**Table 2**).

Because of serious side effects associated with each category of medications, it is imperative for the psychiatric nurses to be familiar with these agents and order diagnostic studies unique to side-effect profiles associated with these agents before initiation. As previously discussed, medical clearance is imperative to rule out physical and substance use disorders that mimic symptoms of bipolar disorders. Periodic (3–6 months) laboratory tests are recommended for safe monitoring of medication levels and metabolic, liver, kidney, and thyroid functioning while taking many of these medication.[30] Equally important is ruling out pregnancy, as mood stabilizers are linked to serious teratonergic side effects. (See Courtney J. Givens: Adverse Drug Reactions Associated with Antipsychotic, Antidepressants, Mood Stabilizers, and Stimulants, in this issue.) The choice of the medications that are used to treat a patient with bipolar disorder is determined by the psychiatric nurse prescriber and based on input from the

**Table 2**
**Medications used to treat bipolar disorders**

| Mood Stabilizers for Acute Depression and Acute Mania in Bipolar Illness | | | |
|---|---|---|---|
| Medication | Indication | Serum Levels | Target Dose |
| Aripiprazole (Abilify) | Mania | 150 and 300 ng/mL | 15–30 mg daily |
| Asenapine (Saphris) | Mania | — | 5–10 mg SL BID |
| Carbamazepine (Tegretol) | Mania | 4–10 μg/mL | 200–1600 mg daily |
| Divalproex (Depakote) | Mania | 50–110 μg/mL | 1000–1500 mg daily |
| Lamotrigine (Lamictal) | Mania | 1.5–10 μg/mL | 25–400 mg daily |
| Lithium | Mania | 0.6–1.2 μg/mL | 900–1800 mg daily |
| Lurasidone (Latuda) | Depression | — | 20–120 mg daily with food |
| Olanzapine (Zyprexa) | Mania | 8–47 ng/mL | 5–20 mg daily |
| OFC Olanzapine/fluoxetine | Depression | — | 6/25–12/50 mg daily |
| Quetiapine (Seroquel) | Depression | — | 400–800 mg daily |
| Quetiapine (Seroquel) | Mania | — | 300 mg daily |
| Risperidone (Risperdal) | Mania | — | 1–6 mg daily |
| Ziprasidone (Geodon) | Mania | — | 40–80 mg BID with food |

*Abbreviations:* BID, twice a day; SL, sublingual.

patient, previous medication responses, history of medication adherence, and coexisting substance use and physical disorders. Although there are various guidelines and algorithms available to guide the clinician's decision making, such as the Texas Medication Algorithm Project, there is no algorithm or guideline that is absolute; that decision is left to the treating provider.

*Psychotherapeutic Interventions*

Although pharmacotherapy is helpful in mitigating acute and long-term symptoms associated with bipolar disorder, they often fail to help the patient attain an optimal level of recovery and quality of life. It is widely accepted that nonadherence to a medication regimen is a serious clinical concern in patients with bipolar disorders. Nonadherence to a medication regimen must be continuously monitored through serum levels and observation for early signs of recurrence. Combined with the long-term negative outcomes associated with treating these complex disorders, it is critical for the psychiatric nurse to collaborate with the patient, family members, and other providers to develop person-centered, strength-based and recovery-focused interventions that integrate pharmacotherapy and psychotherapeutic interventions. There is compelling evidence that indicates that the most evidence-based interventions for the patient with a bipolar disorder include CBT, psychoeducation, family interventions, psychosocial rehabilitation, and cognitive remediation.[23,40]

Primary treatment goals include promoting medication adherence, reducing the stigma of psychiatric treatment, addressing cognitive deficits, improving communication, and learning stress management techniques. Family interventions must also include facilitating healthy family interactions and psychoeducation about the identification of early signs of relapse, the importance of adherence to a medication regimen, and stress management. (See Deborah Antai-Otong: Psychosocial Recovery and Rehabilitation, in this issue.)

## SUMMARY

Mood disorders are common, recurring, and debilitating disorders associated with physical morbidity and mortality. Both unipolar depression and bipolar disorders have a high incidence of coexisting psychiatric, substance use, and physical disorders. Left untreated, individuals with these disorders are likely to have a reduced life expectancy and experience impaired functional and psychosocial deficits and poor quality of life. This report provides a brief overview of clinical symptoms of unipolar and bipolar disorders and reviews evidence-based approaches for treating mood disorders regardless of where the patient enters the health care system continuum. As more of these patients seek help in practice settings, it is critical to quickly assess symptoms and initiate person-centered treatment.

Psychiatric nurses are poised to address the needs of these patients through various approaches. Although the ideal approach for mood disorders continues to be researched, there is a compilation of data showing that integrated models of treatment that reflect person-centered, strength, and recovery-based methods produce positive clinical outcomes.

## REFERENCES

1. American Psychiatric Association. Diagnostic and statistical manual of mental disorders. 5th edition. Washington, DC: Author; 2013.
2. Marcus M, Yasamy MT, van Ommeren M, et al. Depression: a global public health concern. World Health Organization Department of Mental Health and Substance Abuse; 2012. Available at: http://www.who.int/mental_health/management/depression/who_paper_depression_wfmh_2012.pdf. Accessed December 30, 2015.
3. Scott KM, Al-Hamzawi AO, Andrade LH, et al. Associations between subjective social status and DSM-IV mental disorders: results from the world mental health surveys. JAMA Psychiatry 2015;71:1400–8.
4. Kessler RC, Berglund P, Demler O, et al. Lifetime prevalence and age-of onset distributions of DSM-IV disorders in the National Comorbidity Survey Replication. Arch Gen Psychiatry 2005;62:593–602.
5. Jopp DS, Park MK, Lehrfeld J, et al. Physical, cognitive, social and mental health in near-centenarians and centenarians living in New York City: findings from the Fordham Centenarian Study. BMC Geriatr 2016;16:1.
6. Arnone D, McIntosh AM, Ebmeier KP, et al. Magnetic resonance imaging studies in unipolar depression: systematic review and meta-regression analyses. Eur Neuropsychopharmacol 2012;22:1–16.
7. Klengel T, Binder EB. Gene-environment interactions in major depressive disorder. Can J Psychiatry 2013;58:76–83.
8. Kessler RC, Amminger GP, Aguilar-Gaxiola S, et al. Age of onset of mental disorders: a review of recent literature. Curr Opin Psychiatry 2007;20:359–64.
9. Kessler RC, Chiu WT, Demler O, et al. Prevalence, severity, and comorbidity of twelve-month DSM-IV disorders in the National Comorbidity Survey Replication (NCS-R). Arch Gen Psychiatry 2005;62:617–27.
10. Merikangas KR, Akistal HS, Angst J, et al. Lifetime and 12-month prevalence of bipolar spectrum in the National Comorbidity Survey replication. Arch Gen Psychiatry 2007;64:543–52.
11. Azorin JM, Belzeaux R, Kaladjian A, et al. Risks associated with gender differences in bipolar I disorder. J Affect Disord 2013;151:1033–40.

12. Kessler RC, Wang PS. The descriptive epidemiology of commonly occurring mental disorders in the United States. Annu Rev Public Health 2008;25:1–16.
13. Jann MW. Diagnosis and treatment of bipolar disorders in adults: a review of the evidence on pharmacologic treatments. Am Health Drug Benefits 2014;7:489–99.
14. Culpepper L. The diagnosis and treatment of bipolar disorder: decision-making in primary care. Prim Care Companion CNS Disord 2014;16 [pii:PCC.13r01609].
15. Geddes JR, Miklowitz DJ. Treatment of bipolar disorder. Lancet 2013;381:1672–82.
16. Lage MJ, Hassan MK. The relationship between antipsychotic medication adherence and patient outcomes among individuals diagnosed with bipolar disorder: a retrospective study. Ann Gen Psychiatry 2009;8:7.
17. Hansell NK, Wright MJ, Medland SE, et al. Genetic co-morbidity between neuroticism, anxiety/depression and somatic distress in a population sample of adolescent and young adult twins. Psychol Med 2012;42:1249–60.
18. Hamon M, Blier P. Monoamine neurocircuitry in depression and strategies for new treatments. Prog Neuropsychopharmacol Biol Psychiatry 2013;45:54–63.
19. Dutta A, McKie S, Deakin JK. Ketamine and other potential glutamate antidepressants. Psychiatry Res 2015;225:1–13.
20. Grieve SM, Korgaonkar MS, Koslow SH, et al. Widespread reductions in gray matter volume in depression. Neuroimage Clin 2013;3:332–9.
21. Chen C-H, Suckling J, Lennox BR, et al. A quantitative meta-analysis of fMRI studies in bipolar disorder. Bipolar Disord 2011;13:1–15.
22. Favre P, Polosan M, Pichat C, et al. Cerebral correlates of abnormal emotion conflict processing in euthymic bipolar patients: a functional MRI study. PLoS One 2015;10:e0134961.
23. Miziou S, Tsitsipa E, Movsidou S, et al. Psychosocial treatment and interventions for bipolar disorder: a systematic review. Ann Gen Psychiatry 2015;14:19.
24. Townsend J, Altshuler LL. Emotion processing and regulation in bipolar disorder: a review. Bipolar Disord 2012;14:326–39.
25. U.S. Department of Health and Human Services: Substance Abuse and Mental Health Services Administration HHS Publication No. (SMA) 09-4432. CMHS-NSP-0193. 2009. Available at: http://store.samhsa.gov/product/Suicide-Assessment-Five-Step-Evaluation-and-Triage-SAFE-T-Pocket-Card-for-Clinicians/SMA09-4432. Accessed December 27, 2015.
26. Smith CJ, Britigan DH, Lyden E, et al. Interunit handoffs from emergency department to inpatient care: A cross-sectional survey of physicians at a university medical center. J Hosp Med 2015;10:711–7.
27. McPeak KE, Sandrock D, Spector ND, et al. Important determinants of newborn health: postpartum depression, teen parenting, and breast-feeding. Curr Opin Pediatr 2015;27:138–44.
28. Betts KS, Williams GM, Najman JM, et al. Maternal depressive, anxious, and stress symptoms during pregnancy predict internalizing problems in adolescence. Depress Anxiety 2014;31:9–18.
29. Melrose S. Seasonal affective disorder: an overview of assessment and treatment approaches. Depress Res Treat 2015;2015:178564.
30. American Psychiatric Association. Practice guidelines for the treatment of patients with major depressive disorders. 3rd editon. Arlington (VA): American Psychiatric Association; 2010.
31. Trivedi MH, Rush AJ, Wisniewski R, et al. Evaluation of outcomes with citalopram for depression using measurement-based care in STAR*D: implications for clinical practice. Am J Psychiatry 2006;163a:28–40.

32. McIntyre RS, Filteau MJ, Martin L, et al. Treatment-resistant depression: definitions, review of the evidence, and algorithmic approach. J Affect Disord 2014; 156:1–7.
33. Beck JS. Cognitive behavior therapy: basics and beyond. 2nd editon. New York: The Guilford Press; 2011.
34. Cuijpers P, Cristea IA, Ebert DD, et al. Psychological treatment of depression in college students: a metaanalysis. Depress Anxiety 2015. http://dx.doi.org/10.1002/da.22461.
35. Sienaert P. What we have learned about electroconvulsive therapy and its relevance for the practising psychiatrist. Can J Psychiatry 2011;56:5–12.
36. Leiknes KA, Cooke MJ, Jarosch-von Schweder L, et al. Electroconvulsive therapy during pregnancy: a systematic review of case studies. Arch Womens Ment Health 2015;18:1–39.
37. Yuan TF, Li A, Sun X, et al. Vagus nerve stimulation in treating depression: A tale of two stories. Curr Mol Med 2016;16(1):33–9.
38. Dunner DL, Aaronson ST, Sackeim HA, et al. A multisite, naturalistic, observational study of transcranial magnetic stimulation for patients with pharmacoresistant major depressive disorder: durability of benefit over a 1-year follow-up period. J Clin Psychiatry 2014;75:1394–401.
39. Peselow ED, Clevenger S, IsHak WW. Prophylactic efficacy of lithium, valproic acid, and carbamazepine in the maintenance phase of bipolar disorder: a naturalistic study. Int Clin Psychopharmacol 2015. [Epub ahead of print].
40. Gonzalez I, Echeburua E, Liminana JM, et al. Psychoeducation and cognitive-behavioral therapy for patients with refractory bipolar disorder: a 5-year controlled clinical trial. Eur Psychiatry 2014;29:134–41.
41. Centers for Disease Control and Prevention. Suicide among adults Aged 35–64 Years–United States, 1999–2010. MMWR Morb Mortal Wkly Rep 2013;62:1–24. Available at: http://www.cdc.gov/mmwr/preview/mmwrhtml/mm6217a1.htm. Accessed December 27, 2015.

# Index

*Note:* Page numbers of article titles are in **boldface** type.

Nurs Clin N Am 51 (2016) 353–366
http://dx.doi.org/10.1016/S0029-6465(16)30010-X
0029-6465/16/$ – see front matter

# *Moving?*

## *Make sure your subscription moves with you!*

To notify us of your new address, find your **Clinics Account Number** (located on your mailing label above your name), and contact customer service at:

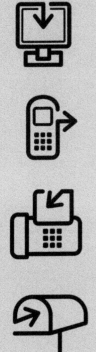

**Email: journalscustomerservice-usa@elsevier.com**

**800-654-2452** (subscribers in the U.S. & Canada)
**314-447-8871** (subscribers outside of the U.S. & Canada)

**Fax number: 314-447-8029**

**Elsevier Health Sciences Division**
**Subscription Customer Service**
**3251 Riverport Lane**
**Maryland Heights, MO 63043**

*To ensure uninterrupted delivery of your subscription, please notify us at least 4 weeks in advance of move.

Printed and bound by CPI Group (UK) Ltd, Croydon, CR0 4YY

03/10/2024

01040390-0002